THE STUD MUFFIN

A Novel

By

Don P. Pendergrass

This book is a work of fiction. Places, events, and situations in this story are purely fictional. Any resemblance to actual persons, living or dead, is coincidental.

ISBN: 1-4107-7343-4 (e-book)
ISBN: 1-4107-7342-6 (Paperback)

Library of Congress Control Number: 2003094773

This book is printed on acid free paper.

Printed in the United States of America
Bloomington, IN

1stBooks – rev. 09/04/03

ACKNOWLEDGEMENTS

Thanks to Margo Maxwell and Melinda Turner for their time and help critiquing my novel. Special thanks go to my children, Karen, Laurie Ann, and Jake for all their input and help. Very special thanks to Dr. Sim Shattock for his help and editing my novel. I would be remiss not to express my sincere gratitude to my ex wife, Tina, for the criticism and encouragement she gave.

A NOTE FROM THE AUTHOR

Being a trucker most of my life I would like to leave these thoughts to the reader. Just about every thing you own or have but your soul and conscience was brought to you by a trucker. Next time a truck gets in your way—remember this—that trucker could be bringing you something else. Cut 'um some slack.

Chapter 1

"Please don't let this be what I think it is," Leon said to himself shining his flashlight on the figure lying in the grass. Cautiously nudging what he at first thought was a discarded statue with his tire bumper, ice shards fell to the fresh mown grass from the corpse's ear. Colored the shade of a fryer packed in ice (probably a shade bluer), the naked man lay frozen staring into nothingness out of wide-open ice-glazed eyes. Steamy fog is oozing from the frozen man like an open freezer door on a hot summer afternoon. Looking at the man lying on his left side with his knees pulled up to his stomach, his arms hugging his legs below the knees, his body forever frozen as if he had sat down to rest a moment and fallen over, Leon's own body began to tremble.

"Son of a bitch," said Leon, shaking his head, instantly regretting using profanity. He hadn't used those words since high school. Leon Sizemore was not a typical long-haul trucker. Born and raised in a strict Pentecostal family in Covington County near Opp, Alabama, Leon was thirty-one, married, and the father of two girls. A devout Pentecostal, he had never tasted an adult beverage, never tasted tobacco, or never dated another woman other than his wife. Clean-shaven, shorthaired, five-foot-nine, Leon was a great looking guy with impeccable manners. He didn't have that bronckey know-it-all attitude that most long-haul truckers usually acquire after a few years on the road.

Rolling eastbound on I-10 in South Louisiana Leon had needed to make a pit stop. Ordinarily he would never have exited at the Butte

Larose exit, but his bladder changed his mind. The Butte Larose exit is off the seventeen-mile long twin-span bridge across the Atchafalaya River Basin Swamp between Baton Rouge and Lafayette, Louisiana. This exit has a huge rest area for four wheelers beneath the twin-elevated bridges as well as the exit for Louisiana Highway 31. In contrast to all other rest areas in Louisiana, traffic in both directions use the same common rest area under the twin elevated bridges. A public boat-launching ramp is on the west end of the rest area and the Atchafalaya River levee is the east boundary.

After doing his business on the shoulder of the exit ramp near the stop sign, Leon's curiosity handed him the situation he was in. He just had to walk out there across that newly mown grass in the edge of the shadows, mostly to stretch his legs and see what somebody had thrown out. Now here he was standing over a frozen dead man on a hot and humid August night in the middle of the Atchafalaya River Swamp, mosquitoes vampiring every square inch of his exposed skin as he alternately scratched his head and ass trying to make up his mind what to do next. Dreading making that call, Leon knew it had to be made. If his load of ground beef patties were late he would just have to deal with the meat folks when he got to Harahan.

Leon walked back to his big truck and climbed up in the cab. Dialing *LSP, Leon reported his discovery to a skeptical trooper in Lafayette.

Answering the phone at Troop I Headquarters of the Louisiana State Police unit in Lafayette, Trooper Elwin Landry drank his third cup of coffee as he listened to Leon tell him what he had found at the Butte Larose exit. Trooper Landry was in no mood tonight to listen to drunks and dopeheads that call in prank calls. Taking his name and instructing Leon to remain where he was until a trooper showed up, Elwin turned to another trooper hanging out in the dispatch room and said, "Dis is da best of the week here, Aaron."

"Say what?"

"Dis trucker says he done found a man froze solid as a rock out dere at da Butte Larose rest area east bound. Man, I just ain't in the mood to listen to dis shit tonight, bro. I'm gonna call Cecil and tell him to go ahead and check it out. He just reported that he was at Henderson, but I need you to haul ass out dere and if dis ain't exactly what dis trucker said it is, bring his ass in."

2

"You know I can't tell Cecil what to do if he don't wanna bring that dude in. He outranks me and I done made dat mistake already," said Trooper Aaron Juneaux getting ready to leave.

"I'll tell him. Get on out dere," answered Elwin turning to call Sergeant Cecil Bell.

Already sleepy at ten-thirty, Cecil had stopped in Henderson for coffee after turning a vanload of Mexicans loose with one headlight, a hard copy ticket, and a severe ass chewing. He answered the call and headed to the Butte Larose exit. Putting an extreme belly stretching on the taxpayers Crown Victoria police cruiser, Trooper Bell was there in minutes and found the truck his dispatcher had described.

Trooper Bell got out with flashlight, portable radio in hand, unsnapped the safety strap on his pistol holster, and approached Leon's rig. As Trooper Bell approached Leon got out of the truck and waited until Cecil asked, "Are you Leon Sizemore?"

"Yes sir," answered Leon handing the trooper his CDL.

"You called in about a man froze to death?"

"Yes sir."

"Where is he?"

"Back here behind my trailer, officer," said Leon turning and walking toward the back of the trailer as Cecil walked along with him.

Trooper Bell ignored his dispatcher's call on the portable radio as he knelt to examine the dead man. Fog was still rising from the man as the trooper carefully examined the corpse and the area around him noting that Leon was standing ten feet away.

Trooper Bell looked up at Leon indicating that they return to the trooper's cruiser.

Not wanting to put his findings on the radio, Cecil told Leon to stand near the back of the cruiser until he made a call to dispatch from his cell phone.

Cecil carefully explained what he had found. Trooper Landry asked, "What does that trucker have to say about it?"

"I haven't questioned him yet, Elwin. Send a deputy to bring the coroner and dispatch an ambulance out here. Call the Captain and tell him what's going down out here. He needs to get out here fast. This situation is too big for me and you to handle."

"I ain't calling da Captain, Cecil. I ain't about to get my ass chewed out for waking him up."

"I said call the Captain," said Trooper Cecil Bell cutting off Elwin and clearly pulling rank at the same time.

"Okay, but he ain't gonna like being called out."

"Don't worry about it, I'll take the flack," answered Cecil pressing the disconnect button, clipping the phone to his holster belt, and getting out his tape recorder and laying it on his clipboard.

Turning and walking towards Leon, Cecil said, "Tell me how you come about finding this man, Mr. Sizemore. I'm going to record all of our conversation, okay?"

"Okay," said Leon nodding in agreement.

"Why did you stop here?"

"I needed to use the restroom."

"Where you from?" asked Sergeant Bell looking at his CDL.

"Opp, Alabama."

"That your truck?"

"Yes sir."

Other than Leon's being overly nervous, Trooper Bell was satisfied that Leon was only reporting what he had found and was in no way involved. Trooper Bell did ask Leon not to leave until his boss got there and asked some more questions.

Minutes later Trooper Aaron Juneaux showed followed by a convoy of parish deputies from Lafayette and Iberville. Cecil quickly dispatched the deputies to seal off all exits and entrances to the rest area.

"No one will be allowed to leave unless I have personally interviewed them. I want to know every person's name and address in this rest area, at the boat ramps and parked on the shoulder of the road, and if any boats are tied up at the dock across the levee I want to talk to them as well," ordered Trooper Bell.

"Most all these folks are asleep in their cars, Cecil," remarked one of the Lafayette Parish deputies.

"Wake their asses up, bro. These people ain't supposed to be camping out here in the first place. Anybody that is not cooperative, bring them to me. Start with the truckers first, but question every single person here," said Trooper Bell.

Lafayette and Iberville sheriff dispatchers had ordered all available units to the Butte Larose rest area. Lafayette and Iberville sheriff departments worked well in tandem at night, especially in the Butte Larose area. Shortly, plenty of officers were there to help and do a little rubber necking. All officers were quickly assigned to questioning every occupant in the rest area and down at the boat launching ramps on the far west end of the rest area.

Deputy Theottis Desmeaux walked up to an eighteen-wheeler pulling a reefer trailer almost identical to Leon Sizemore's parked on the shoulder of La. 31, known locally as the levee road. The tractor unit was a red Navistar International 7800 series, running lights on, headlights out, big Pro Sleeper cab, big everything. The unit's big 500 horsepower Detroit Diesel engine idling about 800 rpm pulling the superb air-conditioning unit wringing moisture out of the high humidity air and discharging the condensation to the ground like a mad cow peeing through a pole bridge. The dome light was on inside the cab. A bearded man sat behind the wheel with a clipboard laid on the steering wheel working on his logbook. Theottis walked up and knocked on the door of the big red truck.

"What's the problem, officer?" asked the bearded man as he got out of the truck without being asked and quickly slammed the door.

Theottis noted the quick door slam, indicating that this driver had been in south Louisiana before. The tall bearded driver was not about to let his cab fill up with mosquitoes. "I need to ask you some questions," said Theottis.

"Sure officer. Fire away."

After asking several questions and looking at his commercial driver's license Theottis said, "Would you walk over there with me and talk with the State Trooper in charge, please?"

Nodding in agreement, the driver held up one finger indicating he needed a minute. Opening his truck door and stepping up on the top running board, the driver removed a long-sleeved denim shirt, a black cowboy hat, and flashlight. He slipped the long-sleeved shirt on over his dressy western shirt for mosquito protection, stuck his hat on, and indicated he was ready.

5

Standing under the mercury vapor lights that bathed the whole rest area, Trooper Cecil Bell was issuing orders to everyone in sight, clearly agitated that no one had seen a damn thing. Cecil was again talking to Leon Sizemore asking questions as Theottis and the bearded trucker approached. Waiting for Cecil to pause, the tall bearded trucker lit a cigarette. Cecil turned and said, "Could I bum one of those off of you, bud?"

The bearded truck driver handed him the pack and a lighter. "Been quit five and half years. This is not a good night. Thanks. What'ya got, Theottis?"

"We have an eyewitness here that can tell us how and when the frappé monsieur come to be here," said Theottis, inadvertently naming the case of the frozen man, 'frappé monsieur,' and handing Cecil the bearded trucker's CDL. Not an eyebrow raised as Theottis said, 'frappé monsieur'. Every deputy there spoke Cajun French as a job requirement. Sergeant Cecil Bell was a French-speaking Cajun from Esterwood but never spoke French unless necessary. Cecil used the local English-French dialect only with close friends and family speaking English without a trace of French accent.

Holding the CDL in his left hand and flashlight in the other, Cecil quickly scanned the license as he had thousands over the years and asked, "Raymond L. Cloyd, is this your current address in Brandon, Mississippi?"

"Yes, that is my home address."

"Where is your rig parked?"

"Right over there," answered Raymond indicating the lone big truck in that direction.

"What are you doing here in a rest area for cars?" asked Cecil.

"I'm not in the rest area, officer. I'm parked on the shoulder of the levee road," answered Raymond in a voice that was not Mississippi Redneck.

Noting his voice, appearance, and checking his date of birth Cecil quickly concluded this trucker was ten years younger looking than his fifty-three years.

"Are you a native of Mississippi?"

"Yes, I was born and raised in Mississippi."

"Don't talk like it."

"You don't talk like a Cajun either," said Raymond in a joking sort of way.

Cecil knowing from long experience of dealing with strangers, especially truckers, and quickly reading them, that intimidation would never work on the bearded man standing before him. "How long you been parked out there?"

Looking at his watch, Raymond answered, "Fifty-five minutes."

"What have you been doing all of this time?"

"I parked, got my stuff and walked over to restroom, cleaned up, used the bathroom, and come back out and was doing some paper work."

The commotion over where the corpse lay grew louder, shutting down Cecil's interview with Raymond. The deputies had flagged off the whole area around the frozen man, and the coroner was now walking towards Cecil with three deputies and a trooper.

"Damned if I ever seen anything like this before, Cecil. That ole boy is frozen solid. Somebody must have been really pissed off at that poor bastard about something or he done somebody some real dirt," said Dr. Lance Goudeaux. Dressed in a tank top, shorts, wearing sandals and a planter's straw hat, the coroner had left a pool party at his house and been drinking beer. He was not drunk. Everyone knew that Dr. Goudeaux's reputation was unmatched. His opinion was never questioned.

Dr. Goudeaux's life ambition was to be just like his daddy who was also a doctor. So far, he had lived up to all of his aspirations. Owning a full partnership in a family clinic with his daddy and two more doctors, Dr. Goudeaux was well off financially. A big person for his five-ten frame, two hundred thirty-five pounds, forty-six, great personality, and in prime physical condition. He was married with six children. Out of his office though, Dr. Goudeaux was a world-class womanizer. His dark complexion and great looks often bore fruit with the younger women. His wife didn't seem to care as long as he didn't get her pregnant again.

The one thing Dr. Goudeaux had that intrigued his clients and friends was his unique perception and his uncanny predictions. Cecil listened to the doctor rave on about his theory of the frappé monsieur until he excused himself and pulled a deputy aside, telling him to get the doctor back to his party. Dr. Goudeaux agreed not to discuss this case, especially with the news people, until tomorrow. The deputy had him out of there in minutes.

The TV news crews were allowed into the rest area for the simple reason that they were blocking traffic up on the seventeen-mile long elevated bridge over the Atchafalaya River Basin Swamp. Cecil had them park on the west side of the rest area near the boat launching ramps. A deputy was assigned the task of keeping them there until the preliminary investigation was done. Cecil promised them a shot of the body before it was moved.

Raymond and Leon were still standing around waiting for Trooper Bell to finish his questioning. Shortly, Sergeant Bell returned and asked, "Mr. Cloyd, please tell me what you saw concerning this matter."

"Before I answer, did I see a murder or someone dumping a body?"

"You don't know what was dumped out there on the grass, Mr. Cloyd?"

"From what I have gathered is that somebody has dumped a frozen man over there, and I saw them do it but didn't know what they dumped. Am I close?"

"Yeah, that's about it Mr. Cloyd."

"Could I have a look at the corpse?"

Hesitating for a moment, Sergeant Bell answered, "Sure, why not?"

Raymond turned on his flashlight as he stooped down to examine the corpse. Raymond closely checked the dead man's face, back, legs and as much of his stomach as he could see. Raymond then checked the corpse's hands and fingertips. He quickly rolled the dead man over on his other side before Cecil could object. Carefully searching for a bullet hole or some clue that the dead man may have been killed then frozen. Raymond stood up and faced Cecil.

"Well?"

"This man was frozen while he was alive, Sergeant Bell. Stripped naked and then frozen to death."

"Just how'n the hell do you know that?" asked Cecil.

"Look at his fingernails and hands. They were a bloody pulp before he froze."

"I see what you're talking about. Must have tried to claw his way out before he died, huh?"

"That's the way I see it."

"Man, what a hell of way to die."

"Yeah, that coroner was right about one thing."

"What's that?"

"This dude has really pissed somebody off, big time."

"Could I ask you a question, sort of off the record?" said Trooper Bell, pulling Raymond out of earshot off the other officers hanging on to every word spoken so far.

"Have you ever worked with a coroner or in the medical field?"

"Yeah, in Vietnam I was assigned to a MASH Unit and wrote up the cause of death for the doctors in the unit. I done two tours over there doing the help the doctor thing, writing up the reports, and bagging bodies."

"Okay, tell me what you see here."

"Whatcha mean, officer?"

"If you were writing up a report what would you say?"

Walking back to the corpse and shining his flashlight down at the frappé monsieur, Raymond carefully choosing his words replied, "I see a white male, naked, frozen solid, in a sitting position hugging his legs to his chest. It is my observation that this person was frozen alive due to the condition of his hands and fingernails. This man is probably twenty-five to thirty years old, slim athletic build, well groomed and clean-cut."

"Okay, now tell me exactly what you saw. Try to remember every detail. I'm recording your statement."

"After I pulled in the rest area and cleaned up, I returned to my rig and was doing some paperwork. This big ole red two bedroom (extra-large sleeper cab) Pro Sleeper International tractor 'bout like mine pulling a reefer trailer drops off the west bound git off ramp into the rest area and parks about where that truck is sitting," indicating the spot that Leon's big KW now occupied.

"What happened next?"

"The dome light comes on in the International and this woman was all over the driver the minute he pops the brakes. This ole gal was something else, nothing on above her waist. Boy, did she have a set of hooters and was rubbing 'em all over the driver's face. The driver opened a can of beer, she took it out of his hand, and she took a big long drink and went back to teasing the driver. He turns off the dome light and they both get in the sleeper."

"So the trucker scores with a woman with big hooters, that figures."

"Not quite, officer."

"What you mean by that?"

"Well, I started on my paperwork again and not ten minutes later the woman turns on the dome light. This heifer is sitting in the driver seat dialing a cell phone. In less than a minute a new four-door gray Ford pickup pulls in front of the International, and a man and woman get out and the gal in the International gets out, and they talk a minute. They all go to the back of the trailer. The man takes a key and unlocks the padlock on the trailer door. He opens the door and they talk a minute. The man then jumps up in the trailer and moves something to the back of the trailer. The older woman goes to the pickup and returns with what looked to me like a horse blanket. She hands the blanket to the guy up in the trailer. He rolls this corpse here, indicating the frozen man, onto the blanket, and drags the corpse to the bumper plate. The girls grab the blanket and ease it to the ground. The man jumps to the ground and all three of them drag this man to where he is now and unceremoniously dumps his dead ass out of the blanket onto the grass. The girls get into the pickup, the guy gets into the big truck, and they all drive off."

"That's it?"

"Yeah, except for two things."

"What's that?"

"That dude drove that truck away like he had drove that rig recently."

"Why you say that?"

"Cause he knew where everything was in the International, no hesitation or fumbling for light switches or anything like that. He pops the head lights on, releases the brakes, and hauls ass."

"Which direction?"

"Westbound."

"What direction did the truck come from when it arrived here?"

"From the west."

"Did the truck have a company name on the door or something?"

"Yeah. It had a great professional lettering job on the doors. I don't remember the name but it was oak something or other Louisiana on the door. Just another red International rig very similar to mine. It was clean with a fresh wash job—you know, shiny wheels, shiny bumper, and all."

"What about the reefer trailer? Anything lettered on it that you noticed?"

"No, not a thing, just an owner-operator version Utility reefer. Aluminum wheels and stainless steel doors, forty-five footer. Must've been a chicken-hauler."

"Why?"

"If he hauled garbage (produce) from the West Coast he would more than likely have a forty-eight foot spread axle like mine."

"What's the other thing you mentioned?" inquired Trooper Bell carefully watching Raymond's body english and demeanor.

Knowing the trooper was still profiling him, Raymond looking directly into the trooper's eyes answered in a soft voice audible only to Trooper Bell, "They wanted this guy to be found, Officer Bell. They had to know I was watching them with me sitting over there with my dome light on in my truck. I was going over to see what it was they dumped but this other driver beat me to it. They were looking and watching but dumped the guy anyway. You see what I'm saying?"

Trooper Bell nodded his head indicating they walk toward his rig. Out earshot of the other officers, Sergeant Bell said, "Yeah, I see what you're talking about. I guess that truck was probably stolen and drove over here by some drug thugs."

"Looking back on the whole deal I witnessed, I doubt that theory."

"Every time the drug thugs put someone down they want to make a statement."

"That's true but in this case these two women were helping. Them women didn't look like users at all to me, officer. These were just regular-looking folks that's making a statement bout something else is my hunch."

"Like what?"

"Try stealing, rape, adultery, and making it a real stretch, child molestation or something like that. Think about it officer: drug thugs ain't gonna drop a body off in a rest area full of folks and expose themselves to a potential eyewitness. Think about it."

"You've been a great help, Raymond. Do you have a cell phone?"

"Yeah, I sure do," said Raymond digging a business card out of his shirt pocket and handing it to the trooper.

"I will call you if I think of any more questions," said the trooper handing Raymond his CDL.

"Yeah, be glad to help anyway I can."

As the bearded trucker walked back to his rig, Cecil watched him a minute, thinking, "That man would have made one hell of a good crime scene investigator."

Chapter 2

On Oakwood High School prom night fourteen years ago in a pickup on a secluded oilfield road, a girl child was conceived by Lea Hart. Milt Myers was the conceiver, classmate, and fiancé of Lea. They had planned to be married in the summer, but both sets of parents insisted that they go to college. The teenagers had other plans.

Both Lea and Milt were the only children in two of Oakwood's most successful and respected business families. The Myers was long haul trucking and logging contractors; the Harts were prominent realtors in southwest Louisiana and southeast Texas in the greater Golden Triangle area. Beaumont, Orange, and Port Arthur, Texas and all the smaller towns in the area even lapping over into Louisiana are known as the Golden Triangle

When Lea told her mom that she was pregnant and she and Milt were getting married—the shit hit the fan. The tirade was short lived, Lea's mom remorsefully remembered that she herself and her husband had thought she was knocked up and had eloped, later finding out she was not pregnant. Sue Hart simply hugged her daughter, assuring her everything would be all right.

A church wedding was quickly arranged. Oakwood, a small town only twelve miles from the Texas line, was full of day counters. The busybody day counters would actually mark the wedding day and then mark off nine months to ascertain if hanky panky had occurred before the wedding vows. The busybody day counters were a bit disappointed. Lea's term was a little long. By the very best dead reckoning, the busybodies conceded that the baby was probably conceived on the honeymoon night, saving the reputation of the newlyweds from the scandal the small-town busybodies loved to spread.

Roger Hart, Lea's dad, found the newly weds a nice little house on twelve acres near the Myers home just out of town a couple of miles. Milt went to work for his dad full time. Lea and Mia Comeaux, Lea's best friend since kindergarten, enrolled in a cosmetology school in nearby Lake Charles.

Mia quickly decided that she wanted a different career. She dropped out of the cosmetology school and enrolled at Lamar University in Beaumont. Working for the Harts in their real estate office in Beaumont part time and graduating in business management, Mia's second career choice was perfect for her. Lea simply dropped out three weeks later and went home to have her baby and take care of Milt.

Eight pounds and three ounces, a fairly easy delivery, Sly Myers was born into a family devoted to giving her the very best of everything. Both grandmothers objected to the name Sly. Lea overruled all objections.

A beautiful baby when she was born, Sly, now fourteen, is a stunningly beautiful young girl. Tall, nearly as tall as her mom, five nine and a half inches, coal black hair, aqua blue eyes, and a figure any grown woman would kill for. Sly's aqua blue eyes, black hair, and olive complexion were exquisite. Sly had it all, the looks, the figure, complexion, outgoing personality, and poise of a twenty-two year old woman.

Sly had won every beauty contest she had entered. She was the product of doting parents and grandparents who had the means to get and give anything to make her beautiful and happy. Appointments— dentist and orthodontist, lessons—piano lessons, dance lessons, poise lessons, and karate lessons used most of her free time in the afternoons. Her parents, grandparents, and Aunt Mia were unrelenting with their demands on Sly for perfection.

Sly, quite an athlete, played softball, basketball, soccer, and volleyball. She did go to cheerleaders camp and was now a cheerleader for Oakwood High School football team. Her parents and godmother, Mia Comeaux, and grandparents saw that Sly never missed a ball practice, appointment, or lesson. Mia and Sly's mom always made sure she wore the latest fashions for teenage girls and her hair was the latest style as long as it wasn't off the wall.

Sly had a horse at her granddaddy Myers farm and rode in playdays with her parents. The grown men at the playdays and everywhere else were paying way too much attention to Sly lately to suit Lea and Aunt Mia. A tall beautiful young woman with a 35-25-34 figure is supposed to attract attention from men—all men. Knowing that, Lea and Mia kept a sharp eye out and carefully monitored all of Sly's activities. Sly's wonderful and outgoing personality made the sharp eyeing and monitoring a full time job. She had never met a stranger and loved to talk to people.

Most of all Sly loved to hibernate in her room to play her guitar and sing country and western songs. Her granddaddy Hart had bought Sly a fine concert guitar after he found out about her interest in country music. Sly had taught herself how to play the guitar along with the help of her granddaddy Myers. She loved to listen to the radio, play along, and sing with the country music stars.

Sly's ambition was to be a country music star; everything else was secondary to her, although she kept her ambitions to herself, carefully spoon-feeding her Granddaddy Myers her intention in small doses. Paw, as Sly called her granddad Myers, loved country music, was quite an accomplished musician himself, and readily helped his granddaughter keeping her secret ambition to himself.

A stifling August afternoon, humidity at nearly a hundred percent, Sly had decided not to go swimming. She was in her room listening to the local radio station. A new disc jockey had been recently hired, and all the teenagers in range of the small FM station in Oakwood listened to Ryan Roberts. He laced his program format with mostly country and western and just a tad of rock.

Ryan Roberts sand Toby Nichols migrated to the Golden Triangle from Kansas. Ryan and Toby vacated the small city in Kansas under the cover off darkness again because of Ryan's obsession with young girls. Ryan stood almost six feet tall, brown hair, brown eyes, and very nice-looking young man. Ryan, now twenty-seven had been accused of bedding a fifteen-year-old cheerleader in Kansas who happened to be the football coach's daughter. Ryan was a pedophile, a young pedophile, but a pedophile just the same. Ryan liked them even younger than fifteen when he could find one. Toby was Ryan's engineer and producer. Working together since high school in radio, both men were the same age and graduated from the same high school in Greeley, Colorado. Highly skilled in electronics and computers, Ryan and Toby were a great team in the radio profession.

Black hair and dark eyes, standing five-ten, Toby was also a handsome man. Neither had ever been married nor had ever considered such a move. Ryan's passion for young girls was the exact opposite of Toby. He liked his women at least five years older than himself. Strange as their personal preferences were with the ladies they made a great team working together.

Sanford Leon Brooks, a.k.a. Ryan Roberts would have never been in Oakwood if he had kept his sexual proclivity under control. Ryan would already be big time, a really big time DJ.

Since first airing their afternoon radio show five weeks ago, Ryan and Toby had kicked every afternoon DJ's ass in the Golden Triangle. Knowing a winner, the station owner gave them free hand with their three-hour show. Selling ads on Ryan's show was a snap. Ryan had stacks of CDs to give away as well as free meals from nearly every restaurant in the listening area. Calls to win CD albums, free restaurant meals, and other stuff on Ryan's radio show now numbered into the hundreds every afternoon.

Like every teenager in the radio stations' range, Sly listened until the format strayed from her country and western music interest.

Being a godmother in South Louisiana is a multiple tier honor practiced in several stages of participation according to the wishes of the parents and godchild. Mia Comeaux, Sly's godmother, assumed the ultimate participation role since the moment Sly was born. Holding Lea's hand while in hard labor and never leaving her friend's since side during Sly's birth, Mia was simply fortifying a relationship close as identical twins, maybe even closer. Aunt Mia to Sly, Mia tactfully involved herself in every facet of raising Sly without infringing on Lea's mother-daughter relationship.

Mia had never married after being jilted when a junior in college. She never had a serious relationship again. Five-seven, naturally dark complexion, black hair that shone a reddish glow in the light. Slim and trim figure on a one hundred and twenty-seven-pound frame, heads always turned when she walked. Her beautiful face and dark, almost black eyes, toothpaste commercial teeth, great never-met-a-stranger personality gave her quite an edge over any woman in the eligible bachelorette department. Fun loving and a party girl, Mia enjoyed being single.

She was also a real estate agent for Lea's parents and got the job by accident. She made a big sale to a hard to please client one Saturday morning while working part time for the Harts and going to college. Because the Harts were too busy to show a house to this cranky client, Mia showed it and sold it, launching a great real-estate selling career. Living high on the hog, pulling in close to two-hundred grand a year, Mia worked out of the Beaumont office, selling in Texas and Louisiana.

Living on the outskirts of Oakwood, Mia never let anything or anybody interfere with being there for Sly. Every other Saturday morning Mia, Lea, and Sly always went shopping and had lunch. Mia and Lea had established this ritual in high school. Sly had made these Saturday excursions a threesome for fourteen years.

Lea Myers and Mia were not supposed to be friends. Two great-looking women usually are never friends for any extended length of time because of jealousy and competition. Lea, a slender five-ten, dishwater blonde, real outdoors suntan, long legged, hazel eyes, great teeth, and her bust almost outsized, if not for her height. Her longish oval face with a distinct jaw line, disturbingly fine lips below a distinctly sculptured nose put Lea up there in the Mrs. America category. Mia and Lea were never in competition for anything. Both women worked hard at being beautiful. Both were successful. If one of them made it known to the other what her desire was the other simply went all out to help the other obtain her wish.

Lea's husband Milt, stout built and same height as his bride, was a hundred and eighty pound sandy-haired guy. Milt was now a full partner with his dad. Lea was a full time mom and bookkeeper for the company.

Listening to the radio, Sly was sure she knew the answer to a trivia question about a country singer. She dialed and was lucky enough to be the twelfth caller and correctly answered the question. Nearing the end of the program Ryan, still on the air, told her to come to the station the next day to get her CD. Playing another record, he kept Sly on the phone and suggested that if she wanted to she could come by his apartment and pick it up in about an hour. When he gave her his address, she decided to ride her bike over and pick up her CD. Mom had driven to Mam Maw and Paw Myers to ride her horse and would be gone a couple of hours. Ryan and Toby had rented an apartment from the Harts about a mile from her house back toward town.

Forty-five minutes later, wearing white shorts, yellow halter-top, and tennis shoes with no socks, Sly knocked on Ryan's door. Hearing loud music inside, she was about to knock again when the door opened.

Holding the door open, Ryan seemed younger than twenty-seven and quite a hunk, just as the girls at school had described him. He gave Sly the once over. Wearing only a pair of gym shorts, hair still wet from showering, a faint aroma of a great-smelling after-shave lotion, smiling, showing a great set of teeth, Ryan introduced himself saying, "Hi, I'm Ryan. You must be Sly?"

"Hi, yes I am. Nice to meet you," answered Sly.

"Would you care to come in? I'll get your CD for you."

"No, not really, I am in a hurry," said Sly noticing him again giving her the once over, and not even trying to be discreet in his staring. Sly, remembering what her mama and Aunt Mia told her regularly, "Never ever let yourself get into a place where a grown man can isolate you." Her Aunt Mia only last week told her in detail what some grown men would do to her if she happened to let herself get into situation where they were isolated from other people. Aunt Mia told her she was too young to even think about sex yet.

Sly, looking Ryan over was not remembering the last part Aunt Mia told her. Looking at Ryan's hairy chest and legs suddenly sent fire and spasms throughout her entire body. She could tell he had on no underwear under the flimsy shorts. Noting the bulge, she wondered if was he purposely exposing himself or was just endowed?

"Come in and drink a soda, Sly. It must hot riding that bike."

"Well, maybe just for minute," she answered as she walked into his apartment.

Shutting the door and heading for the fridge, Ryan filled two styrofoam cups with ice and soda from a two-liter bottle. Sly sipped the soda as she looked the apartment over. No pictures were on the living room, kitchen, and dining area walls.

"What do you do besides riding around Oakwood on your bike collecting CDs, Sly?"

"I like to ride my horse, go swimming, play softball, and play my guitar and sing."

"Bet you like rock?"

"No, I hate it, I like country music," answered Sly, carefully choosing her words and cocking her head slightly. She smiled and flirted just as she had watched her Aunt Mia do with men since she was old enough to pay attention. Aunt Mia could make men stammer and uncomfortable with her smile and innuendoes. Sly was getting a real rush watching a grown man whose profession was speaking stumble for words as his eyes groped her body. She was out of her league here, Ryan was no bumbling high school football jock but a real grown hunk twice her age knowing exactly where every button was and exactly when to push the button.

"I am gonna be a country music star. I've written a couple of great songs," continued Sly. "I play my guitar and sing, never played for anyone but my granddaddy though."

"I would like to hear a future country music star play and sing. If you are good enough I know people in the business that can get you an audition," said Ryan, wasting no time, he was too close to her before she realized he was there. As he invaded her space, she moved back only to find herself cornered between the kitchen bar and wall. Ryan rubbed her shoulder and it felt so good. She looked him in the eye and knew it was time to go. He was already getting worked up as he stepped closer and intentionally brushed his crotch against her thigh. His manhood had come alive as he rubbed it on her thigh and ran his hand down her back to her halter straps.

Sly deftly grabbed his hand and asked, "Could I have my CD, Ryan? I am leaving."

Ryan softly replied, "You just got here Sly. Stay and we will have some fun."

"I'm outa here," said Sly as she pushed past him and had the door open before he could react. "Where is my CD?"

"Here it is, right here," said Ryan as he unzipped a cloth briefcase sitting in the chair, fumbled for a second or two and handed her a CD.

"Why don't you come down to the radio station and let me cut you a demo CD?" If it's good, I know who to send it to. I can help you with your singing career

"Thanks, Ryan," said Sly as she turned and walked to her bike, straddled it and rode off toward her house leaving him standing in the door.

"She will be back," he said to himself, "They all come back for this," as he rubbed his crotch smiling.

Across the street down two houses a blue haired day counter stood on her porch with broom in hand shaking her head saying to her broom, "They starting younger and younger this day and time. Used to start about sixteen. That girl is barely fourteen."

Thinking about Ryan and her reaction to him gave Sly a very guilty feeling and at the same time a feeling of great accomplishment. She had gotten an offer to help her get started fulfilling her dream. She had to admit to herself that she was attracted to the man knowing that was an absolute no-no from the word go. She liked the way he smelled, the way he touched her, and best of all, his offer to help her. Sly knew that if she asked him to help her that he would expect sex in return, not that it wouldn't probably be great, but sex was out of the question.

Sleepless that night, Sly finally decided to call Ryan and ask him to cut a CD. If she were professional enough he would encourage or discourage her. She would insist that others be present at the radio station when she auditioned for him. It would be nice to have a CD to play for her parents, Aunt Mia, and her friends.

Sly called the next afternoon and set up the audition for Saturday morning at nine-thirty. Ryan assured her that others would be at the radio station working including his friend Toby to help him. She made a point of telling Ryan that under no circumstances would hanky-panky be allowed, period. He agreed, thinking no from young girls usually meant yes, especially if they called him back.

Saturday morning, guitar case strapped across her back, Sly rode her bike the two miles into town to the radio station located on the outskirts of town on the Beaumont highway. Needing a fresh coat of paint, the cinder block building housing the radio station set back off the highway enough to have lot of parking space. An ancient live oak with moss hanging like tinsel on a Christmas tree hogged the west side of the lot with its limbs nearly touching the ground. This massive oak was full-grown when Rene' Robert Cavelier claimed Louisiana for France in 1682.

Leaning her bike against the wall of the building under the handicapped parking zone sign, Sly dressed in jeans, pale yellow western cut blouse, and Reeboks with anklets strode into the reception room of the radio station. No one was at the desk. Panic set in but three cars were on the parking lot. After all, it's Saturday and the receptionist is probably off today. She turned to her left, behind a big plate glass window a woman wearing earphones sat in a plush high back office chair surrounded by a console on three sides. She could hear the station's music over the superb sound system that surrounded her as she waited to be noticed by the woman behind the plate glass window.

Ryan casually walked into the reception room saying, "Hi Sly. Ready to cut that big demo?"

"Hi, I guess I'm ready as I'll ever be," answered Sly.

"Come down here with me and let's get started. Toby has us all set up and ready to go," said Ryan noticing her guitar case slung across her back thinking, "Man, I will have to listen to a least an hour of this crap before I can even approach this chick. Will it be worth it?"

Small but very carefully laid out, the recording studio was used primarily to make commercials. Open floor space was at a premium here.

Toby, sitting behind a huge control panel was quickly introduced. Sly's poise, natural beauty, and charm sent up the red flag with a Jolly Roger flying above it. Toby had seen and felt the results of Ryan's escapades with young girls. Toby knew right off that this girl was no slut, juvenile brat, or dope head like most of the girls he messed with. He could tell from her looks and the way she dressed that this one was definitely a no-no for everyone. This one would get a man in the penitentiary or beat to death.

Toby asked if she would like a stool to sit on while she performed and received a "No, I prefer to stand," answer.

Sly sat her guitar case down on the floor and popped the latches. She removed one of the finest Fender Grand Acoustic concert guitars either man had ever seen and they were around country music and rock stars a great deal.

"Hey, that's some kind of a nice guitar you have there, Sly," said Toby rubbing his neck knowing well that usually only the very best professional pickers own an instrument like she had strapped around her neck.

"Yeah, my grandpa bought it for me last year. I like it lots better than my old one."

"What song you want to play and sing, Sly"?

"Grandpa and I wrote this one. We just put the finishing touches on it last weekend. Want to hear it?" asked Sly, strumming her guitar.

"Sure, let'er rip. Ready over there Toby?" asked Ryan, dreading having to listen to another wanna be just to have his way with her later. "Worth every minute of it."

Getting a thumb up from Toby, Ryan nodded his head indicating to Sly to fire away.

Sly played a short intro to her song. He had to admit she was an accomplished guitarist. When she started to sing the small room resonated with a voice like neither man had ever heard. Very distinctive, clear, and easy to follow, Ryan was not particularly listening to the words or music. He was listening to this strikingly distinctive contralto voice, a voice no professional had ever heard before, and a voice he never knew existed. Young as he was, Ryan immediately knew great talent when he heard it.

Sly, finishing her song, looked at Ryan expecting to see jubilation, saw a totally different man staring at the wall, brow furrowed, jaw clinched staring at a spot above the window overlooking the main studio where he and Toby worked each afternoon. Standing there for what seemed forever, though only a couple of minutes passed, Sly began to think they were playing games with her.

Finally, Ryan without looking away from his spot on the wall with his index finger extended gave one complete spin of his right hand. Immediately Sly heard herself on the speakers. Ryan, never looking away from his spot on the wall, shut his eyes and nodded to the rhythm of Sly's song as he listened intently as the speakers played a future number one country hit. Toby, awestruck and dumbfounded,

22

gazed at Sly knowing that he and Ryan had just discovered country music's next superstar.

As the song played down Ryan chopped the ending off with the chop from his right hand and motioned Toby to restart the CD again. All three of them listened again until the last chord was struck. Ryan sitting there staring at the spot above the window and Toby looking out the window, it got so quiet in the recording studio that a mouse peeing on cotton would have sounded like a class five hurricane.

Ryan was not thinking about how and when he would seduce Sly. He was not thinking about how her nipples would be pink and hard or how he could make her beg him to penetrate her virginity. Shutting out every thing, he could see the world's most beautiful teenager dressed in a sequined western outfit on concert stage with her pants leg slit high enough to get that job done.

Ryan could already visualize triple platinum albums, white limos, huge sellout concerts, and money rolling in by the bale. He intended to be her agent and get his share. It was his right to share in her success. After all, he had just discovered the woman that would put all other female country artists on the back burner.

Sly, watching Ryan's every move, glanced at Toby. He was busy burning more CDs but looked up at Sly and gave thumbs up. Ryan finally turned to Sly and said; "We are going to listen to this a couple of more times, Sly. I want to get it in my mind exactly how we want to cut this in a recording studio, with a band or with just you."

"Does this mean that my song has potential?" asked Sly.

"To be honest with you, Sly it is one of the best songs I have ever heard. We are probably going to release this song without a backup band. By the way, did you or your granddad write this song?"

"Paw and I wrote it together."

"It is a great song. I really like it. Could you play another song for us? Do you have any more songs that you and your granddad wrote?"

"Yeah, but they are not really that good."

"Would you play them for us? All of them, Sly. Play what you like. Toby is going to make you a copy and this will be your first album," said Ryan looking at Toby for reinforcement. Both young men knew their ticket to Music City stood before them.

Sly played a couple of her own songs then played the guitar intro into the present number one county and western hit song by a hugely successful female recording artist. Only the trained ears of professionals like Ryan and Toby could distinguish the intro from one of the finest guitarist in Nashville. Her singing was actually better than the lady with the hit song. Sly never once looked down at her hand as she picked or her long slender fingers as they glided across strings and frets as easily as a master guitarist. This did not escape Ryan or Toby. Neither man could believe their eyes and ears. Never had they seen such natural vocal talent, guitar mastery, and beauty wrapped in one package especially so young. Usually a singer has one maybe two of these gifts, never ever all three. Ryan could already see the huge money rolling in.

"Play that first song again, Toby," said Ryan. "This is it, Sly. This is your debut hit."

Listening to her song one more time, Sly put her guitar in its case and announced it was time for her to leave. Toby gave her a CD with her songs on it. Both men stood and said goodbye as she left the radio station.

Ryan and Toby high-fived and celebrated as soon as Sly left the building. Both men always had Music City ambitions. Ryan and Toby cut six demos to send to Nashville. When they finished the demos and discussed who to send them to Toby turned to Ryan and said in a dead calm voice, "If you get out of line with Sly I'll kill your perverted ass if her folks don't. Sly is our ticket to big time,"

"I want to break her in right, my man," laughed Ryan rubbing his crotch.

Toby grabbed him by shirt collar and shook him. Up in his face nose-to-nose Toby growled, "Touch her and your ass is mine, buddy. Don't even stare, flirt, insinuate or nothing." Shoving Ryan backwards as he released his shirt, "Don't screw up my ticket to Nashville."

Chapter 3

Toby Nichols had seen Mia at the pizza parlor two weeks ago. Infatuated by her looks and personality, Toby made it his business to find out all he could about this beautiful woman. Surprised that she was indeed single, intrigued by the fact that she always had been, he made it his business to get to meet her and ask her for a date. He knew she stopped at the convenience store near the radio station at seven-thirty every morning for a coffee to go. Toby made it a point to be in the store when she arrived two days in a row.

He watched as Mia laughed and joked with everyone while she fixed herself a medium-sized cup with three sugars and a packet of creamer. She stirred the condiments into the coffee exactly six times around and stuck a lid on the styrofoam cup. Mia knew everyone she saw, it seemed to Toby. She was a delight to watch and it was easy to understand why she was the highest-paid real estate salesperson in the area. Professional people, tradesmen, truckers, nurses, deliverymen, and everyone else she knew—Mia made it a point to stop briefly and chat with them. Mia put a new a new dimension on what is now called networking. If a property in her area was going on the market, Mia was there to list it, sell it, or buy it outright.

On the third morning Toby was at the coffeepot watching for the new white-over-tan GMC Yukon that Mia drove. Right on time she pulled up in front of the store, talking on a cell phone, shaking her head as she listened. She reached up, pulled the mirrored sun visor down, and pursed her lips to get her lipstick situated perfectly on those luscious lips.

Stepping out of the Yukon, Mia stopped near the door talking to three young men. From their work clothes, the trio were obviously drywall men on their way to do a job. Toby had prepared a cup of coffee exactly as he had watched Mia fix it two mornings in a row. As she approached the coffee urn he handed the cup of coffee to Mia and replied, "I took the liberty of fixing you this just like you fix it, Mia. I'm Toby Nichols and I wanted to meet you."

"How sweet of you, Toby. I don't believe we have met have we?" asked Mia, turning up the charm, still holding his extended hand, not releasing it. Mia, looking into his eyes, continued, "I've never seen you around. Are you new in town?"

"Been in Oakwood a couple months now. Working at the radio station."

"You must have moved here about the time the new DJ did?"

"Yes, we came to Oakwood together. I'm his producer. We have worked together since high school."

"Great, I enjoy listening to your program although I'm not exactly a teenager. Ryan is really doing a great job. I'm sure he couldn't do it without you. Toby, I have to run," finally releasing his hand and watching his eyes. "Can't be late for work. Nice to meet you."

"I would like to take you out for dinner sometime if you are not involved with someone, Mia."

For a fraction of a moment Mia's brow furrowed. Quickly recovering from Toby's straightforward question, she answered, "Let me think about it, Toby. It's awfully sweet of you to fix my coffee and ask me out," said Mia.

As she walked away, Toby shrugged saying to himself, "Well, I tried. God, what a woman."

Driving to Beaumont, Mia laughed at the thought a man at least five years younger than her would come right out and ask for a date the first time they met. The middle-aged executive types would at least wait and call her later. She didn't date married men, no matter how great looking they were. This Toby guy was really a terrific looking young man, he smelled good, had a great looking tight ass, and was not bashful or cocky. She found her cigarettes and fired one up. She always smoked one with her morning coffee on the commute to Beaumont every morning. She seldom smoked any other time.

Mia thought about Toby, wondering what a younger guy like him could do in bed. If no one had asked her out by Friday maybe she just might take Toby up on his offer. "Why in the hell not? I work my ass off trying to stay attractive to men." He had hair on his chest and was a hunk. "Yeah, I might just give him something like he ain't ever had," said Mia aloud, laughing and already getting aroused just thinking about him.

Toby fixed himself a cup of coffee and drove to his apartment he shared with Ryan. A nearly new green Chevy pickup sat in his parking place. He parked on the street, unlocked the apartment door, and entered. Sitting on the couch was a girl about sixteen, kind of heavy and drinking soda from a styrofoam cup. She looked at him, smiled, and returned to watching TV. In Ryan's bedroom he could hear a girl crying, begging, and pleading with Ryan not to hurt her anymore. Toby heard Ryan mumble something, and the girl came through the door naked with her clothes in her hand held up to her breast, and headed to the bathroom. Ryan stuck his head around the partially opened bedroom door and said, "Come on in, Baby. Let's have some fun."

"No, I don't think so, Ryan. I just brought Marcy by to see you," answered the girl on the couch.

"You are not into having some fun?"

"Sure, but only with my boyfriend."

"Don't know what you are missing."

"Don't want to know."

"See you later," said Ryan giving the door a ride.

Shortly, the naked girl, now fully clothed, came out of the bathroom heading towards the front door. She was softly crying.

"Are you okay, Marcy?" asked the girl on the couch, getting up and leaving with Marcy.

"No, I am bleeding bad. I hope it will stop. God, what am I gonna tell Mama if I have to go to the doctor? Ryan hurt me bad," answered Marcy, now crying aloud.

"How old was that one, Ryan?" asked Toby through the door.

"Don't know. She wasn't quite ready. Probably about thirteen or fourteen. She said she was sixteen but she wasn't."

"How do you know?"

"She was a virgin."

"The hell you say. How did you manage to get her over here this time of the morning?"

"She had to wait until her mom went to work."

"You are going to get shot over them young chicks. Why don't you find yourself a grown woman?"

"I like them young."

"Can't satisfy a grown woman?"

"Yes, I can, but I prefer the young ones. I'm going to get some doughnuts. Want some?"

"No, I'm going to walk downtown and hang out a while."

Mia was busy all day in the office. At four o'clock with her work caught up, she headed for Oakwood. She turned her radio to the Oakwood station and listened to a couple of songs. Ryan was finishing a commercial as he started the song he said, "This one is dedicated to Mia, from Toby, my producer. Here it is just for you, pretty lady."

Mia smiled and thought, "Man this guy will do anything to get attention." She said out loud to the radio, "I like this attention from men no matter how young or old."

Mia drove past the radio station, turning a block later toward her home out on the north side of town. She pulled into her driveway, put her Yukon in park, and quickly checked her appointment book. Thinking about laying up awhile in her Jacuzzi and just kicking back, Mia had almost overlooked Sly's hair stylist appointment. Sly had never been inside a hair stylist shop without Mia. Usually weeks in advance Lea and Mia had decided how Sly's hair would be cut. Mia popped the Yukon in reverse and headed to Lea's house to pick up Sly and her mom.

Lea had on a pair of Wrangler jeans, a western shirt, and sandals, expecting Mia when she drove up the driveway to the house. Lea, looking good in her jeans, really maybe just a little too good for a married woman, called to Sly that Aunt Mia was here.

On the way uptown, Sly showed her mom and Aunt Mia a picture in a magazine of a teenage girl with a haircut she would like to have. Both carefully looked at the picture. Mia looked at Lea; Lea in turn looked at Sly, handing her the magazine back. Sly knew without asking that there would be no new hairstyle for her today. Sly didn't get mad; she was old enough to know that her mom and Aunt Mia were two of the greatest-looking women around. Sly wanted to be just like them, so she remained content to let her Aunt Mia, Miss Amber, and Mom make the hairstyle decisions.

Amber Manning had moved back to the area from California less than three months ago, recovering from severe drug and alcohol addiction. Born and raised twenty miles northeast of Oakwood in a family of three sisters. Amber's dad was a pulpwood logger. He had his own truck and worked by himself cutting shortwood for the paper mill up in Deridder. Truly a one-man pulpwood operation ranks in the top five of all the extreme labor-intensive trades known, making hay hauling, roofing, and roughnecking in the oilfields seem like morning exercise. Amber's dad, Harvey Ray, known to be one of the best in the business, was an extremely conservative man with his money. Harvey Ray refused to hire a swamper (helper) to up his production and make his job safer. His wife and Amber went to the woods after school every day to help him load his truck for delivery to the mill early the next day. Amber hooked tongs or ran the loading winch on her dad's truck. When they got home, it was Amber's job to take down her dad's chain saw, clean the air filter and blow the sawdust off the motor with air, fill the gas tank and chain oil tank, then sharpen the chain. To this very day, not a logger anywhere could beat her filing a saw chain. Amber didn't use a gauge. She filed freehanded.

Out on the front porch watching her mom bushog her daddy's hair one Saturday morning, Amber asked her mom to let her cut her Dad's hair. Not giving a crap what her husband's hair looked like, the burnt-out woman handed Amber not only a pair of scissors and comb but a career that eventually achieved acclaim on every movie studio lot in California. Folks in town and at the papermill asked Harvey Ray if he finally broke down and got a barbershop haircut.

When she was sixteen, Amber was cutting half the girls' and boys' hair in her school and some of her teachers'. The man from the state license office showed up one Saturday morning, raising hell with her mamma and daddy about all this cutting hair without a license.

29

Amber was steadily cutting hair. The porch was full of kids and grownups waiting for a haircut. Harvey Ray and the license man were arguing hot and heavy, Harvey Ray thinking he was going to have to pay a huge fine. Finally, Amber told the license man to sit down in her chair.

"For what?" asked the license man incredulously.

"'Cause that's got to be the worst looking haircut I've ever seen. I'm gonna fix it. Sit down. Won't cost you a nickel."

The license man got a free, great-looking haircut, got them long dark legs rubbed on his thighs, got to feel her up when her parents were not looking, and had that ass back in Amber's chair every three weeks for another freebee. Harvey Ray didn't have to pay a fine and Amber kept right on cutting and styling hair and making herself some money. She finished high school and enrolled in a beautician school in Beaumont. Thrilled to be enrolled in one of the best hairstylist-cosmetology schools in the Deep South, the tall, lanky, dark-complexioned logger's daughter was their star. Amber finished the course and went to work in an upscale salon in Beaumont.

Already a legend in the Golden Triangle, Amber Manning left a huge clientele in Beaumont to advance her career. Amber met and dated a California-based cosmetic salesman. She moved to California with him. While living with the salesman, Amber applied for work in one of the movie studios and was soon one of the most sought-after hairstylist make-up artists on the left coast.

Slowly but surely sucked into the Hollywood vortex of big money, alcohol, drugs, and sex, Amber was spiraling out of control on her way down after only nine years on the West Coast. Getting out of a drug rehab for the second time at the age of thirty-two, she realized it was time for another career move. She simply sold off all of her stuff that wouldn't fit into her car, house and all, and drove home to her Daddy's farm near Deridder to get herself together and start a new life.

Amber was Mia's beautician in Beaumont before she flew the coop with the cosmetic salesman. Mia knew all about Amber's talent and fame, and heard she was back home. Mia made it a point to find her. Getting Amber in business in Oakwood took all of Mia's time and effort for a couple of days. Mia had a beauty salon listed for sale in Oakwood and they struck a deal. In three weeks Amber had more clients than she and two more beauticians could handle. Mia, Lea, and Sly were her first customers. Amber had not touched any drugs since she had returned home. She would go out partying and do some drinking, but that didn't make her a bad girl. That's just the South Louisiana way.

Amber studied the teen hairstyle picture in the magazine that Sly had taken the liberty to show her when she sat down in Amber's chair. No one realized that Amber had one of the original photographs for the cover of this very magazine issue framed and hung on the wall of her office. Mia was talking to an elderly blue-haired lady sitting in the next chair but she had an eye on Sly. Shaking her head no to Amber, Mia approached the chair Sly sat in asking, "Sly, why don't we give this different hairstyle campaign a rest, baby?"

"That's right Sly, give it a rest," said Lea, looking up from a magazine. "Amber don't want to listen to that crap about new hairstyles every time you come in here."

"Wrong. Wrong on all that, Lea. I like fixing new styles. This 'un ain't exactly new. I cut this sucker on one of them dickhead movie producer's teenage daughters nearly two years ago."

"Well, does it still look that bad or what?" asked Sly.

"Nobody said the hairstyle looked bad. We just don't think it would look good on you," said Sly's mom.

"I can fix it about halfway between what you have now and that picture. I'll trim it a good bit shorter than it is now, though. It's gonna make that long neck here look even better," interrupted Amber, laying the magazine in Sly's lap. Running her fingers through Sly's hair while checking her profile in the wall mirror, Amber was clearly taking Sly's side.

"We are not styling her hair to make her look like a West Coast hooker, Amber," said Lea.

"Whoa! Let me tell both of you one damn thing right now. If I say it will look good, it will look damn good. The cut I plan to do is this one except the back. I'm gonna feather this down to nothing with a slight wedge shape." answered Amber grabbing the magazine out of Sly's lap holding the cover up for everyone in the beauty shop to see one of the most stunningly beautiful young women in the world. "I put this cut on this heifer about five months ago just for this shoot. I charged 'em three hundred dollars for this. See. Look here if you think I'm joking." Opening the magazine up and pointing to the cover credits Amber continued, "That's my name right there, Amber Manning, hair stylist, and by God nobody ain't leaving out of here looking like some road whore. Do y'all understand that?"

"Tell it like it is, Amber," said the blue-haired lady in the next chair thoroughly enjoying Amber's tirade.

"Can't we just get her hair cut like we want it cut?" asked Mia.

"You damn sure can, but how come Sly don't get to have just a little bit of input here?" answered Amber.

"She can have some say-so, as long as it is acceptable and becoming to her," said Lea.

"This how you want to look, hon?" asked Amber showing her the magazine cover then holding the magazine up for everyone in the salon to see. The oohs and ahs won.

Sly grinned, searching her mom's eyes for approval. Slowly a smile peeled away the frown. Sly looked at Aunt Mia for support. She got it instantly. Amber high-fived Sly, preparing to make her into a beautiful young lady, one even prettier than the model's picture on the cover of the magazine.

Chapter 4

Toby sat in the ragged-out Corolla in front of the hardware store that was the local agent for Fed Ex in Oakwood. He and Ryan had bought shipping envelopes especially for CDs yesterday in Beaumont. Sly's demos would be delivered to record-company executives by ten-thirty Tuesday morning. Guaranteed. The store opened at eight. Toby waited sipping his coffee he bought at the convenience store earlier. Talking to Mia at the coffeepot for a minute, he still hadn't gotten a no to going out with him. Infatuated with this beautiful woman, Toby still had hope.

As he watched everyone around him hurrying to get to work, Toby's mind wandered to Ryan. He had to make Ryan understand that messing around with young girls was going to get him in serious trouble, jail time probably. He had asked around about Sly. Sure enough, her folks had enough clout to make bad things happen to anyone that messed around with her.

When the man flipped the closed sign in the store window to OPEN, Toby jumped out of the car and launched Sly's singing career. He Fed Exed six copies of Sly's demo to Nashville with a carefully written query and bio in each package. Explicit instructions were enclosed to contact Ryan or Toby because they assumed the roles of agent and manager of Sly without any parental consent signed or orally agreed to. Today they planned to ask Sly's mother to let them kick off Sly's career and sign a standard agent's agreement. Ryan suggested that they ask Sly and her mom to come to the radio station office and sign the papers.

Unknown to both men, Lea had planned to drop by the radio station and thank both men for cutting Sly's demo. When Toby called her later that morning and asked her to drop by before their show started today, Lea readily agreed. Toby hinted to Lea that in a day or two he expected to have some fabulous news for Sly.

Lea, wanting to surprise Milt and Sly's grandparents, decided to invite everyone over for a barbecue tonight and let Sly and Paw do their thing. She was the only one Sly had played the CD for yet. She would invite Mia and Amber. Thinking ahead, Lea knew Sly would need Amber because of her experiences in the entertainment business.

Lea got everyone invited and hurried to the grocery store to get all the stuff she had on a long list. After her mom's offer to come over and help, burgers were upgraded to steak and all the trimmings. Milt promised to be home early and start the grilling. Milt's mom always showed up early to help in the kitchen. Anything concerning Sly was always an all-out event. Tonight would be extra special.

Toby now understood perfectly why Sly was such a beautiful young girl. As Lea walked into the radio station office Toby's eyes nearly popped out of his head when he saw Sly's mother. "This has to be the prettiest woman I've ever seen," said Toby to himself, checking her out good. Lea, wearing just a plain white blouse and jeans, tall as Toby in sandals, didn't miss his admiring appraisal of her. She thought to herself, "This man is on up there with Lynn Howard in the hunk department."

Talking, visiting, and heaping praise on Sly, Lea found both men exceptionally knowledgeable of the music business, as expected. Dominating the conversation, Toby explained the potential of Sly's singing career. Sly listened and watched as Toby wooed her mom, painting pictures of the pleasures and fame she and Sly were about to claim. He never stepped over the line by making an outright pass at Lea, but he explored the limits of Lea's fidelity without her realizing that it was she he was feeling out. Toby asked Lea if she could sing like Sly. The question, while not at all out of line but horribly mistimed and misconstrued, sounded like to Lea that he wanted to explore the possibility of herself trying to upstage Sly. Lea, coming back to reality, replied, "Of course not."

Toby finally broached the subject of him and Ryan being Sly's agent and manager. Lea hesitated a second asking, "Are you talking about being professional managers and agents for my daughter?"

"Yes, we expect to have Sly a recording contract within two weeks if you will agree to letting us represent Sly and sign a contract stating that we are her agents," Ryan answered.

"Before anything is signed I have to talk this over with Milt, my husband, and her grandparents and our lawyer. This is going a little to fast for me," said Lea.

"We want to get Sly's career rolling and take her to the top, Lea. To make it happen we need a signed contract because Sly is a minor. I sent her CD to six major recording companies this morning. I expect to hear from every one of them before Friday. Trust us, Lea. We know how to evaluate talent. We do it every day. Sly's talent will make her rich before she is old enough to have a driver's license and finish high school. None of the top female artist has the looks, her mastery of the guitar, and above all else, her beautiful voice. Please think this over and let's get Sly's music recorded," said Toby enumerating Sly's three essential assets on his fingers as he watched Lea's eyes for favorable reaction.

Lea promised to call them tomorrow morning with an answer. Both men walked Sly and Lea to the front door of the radio station. Toby gave Lea a copy of the standard agent's contract and asked that she and her husband look it over and get back with them.

On the way home Sly asked, "Mom, I got the impression that Toby was coming on to you big time. Did you notice?"

Caught offguard and still giddy that a young hunk like Toby would flirt around with a married woman, Lea blushed. "No, not really, baby. I think he was just being nice. He wants me to sign that contract," answered Lea. "He really wants to be your agent. I guess they see real talent in you."

"You think that daddy will let them represent me?" asked Sly.

"Don't see why not," said Lea, turning into her driveway, noticing that both grandmother's cars were parked in the driveway. Lea jumped out to get the party preparations under way.

Mia called to say that she regrettably couldn't be there. A client had asked to look at a house near Vidor and she would be late getting home tonight. Mia asked Lea what the big deal was, and she told Mia that she would show and tell her Saturday when they went shopping.

Milt showed up just as the ladies were ready for him to start grilling the steaks. Lea's mom, Sue, took it on herself to clean the grill, put in the charcoal, and light it. The coals had burned down just right when Milt put the steaks on. Corn on the cob, seasoned with butter, garlic, and lemon juice and wrapped in aluminum foil would be placed on the perimeter of the grill. In the next few minutes all the guests arrived and were sitting on the patio watching Milt tend the grill. Amber had pulled a chair up beside Paw. She liked to talk to him and pick and carry on with him. Paw knew Harvey Ray, Amber's daddy, from way back when he was a shortwood logger himself. Paw was a regular customer of Amber's. Amber was never out of place anywhere she went. She always fit in with the crowd. Mrs. Hart, also a customer of Amber's, said her mouth was a little potty, but in reality she enjoyed Amber's jokes and tirades as much as anyone else.

Sly had pulled up beside Amber. They had become tight after Amber convinced her mom and Aunt Mia to let her fix her hair like she wanted it to look. Amber asked what the occasion of the party was. Lea told her guests that after dinner she had a surprise for everyone.

Later, after everyone had finished eating, the dishes washed, and the kitchen cleaned up, Lea assembled her guest in the den. She told everyone to listen to the CD she was going to play and tell her who was singing. Everyone listened and looked at each other. Paw and Sly looked and listened acting as if they had never heard the singer. Lea played another song on the CD, but still no one could name the singer. Mam Maw Myers smiled to herself. She recognized Sly's guitar playing.

Lea, having a great time teasing everyone, finally said, "I will show you who is singing and playing."

Paw and Sly got up and got their guitars from Sly's room. In minutes no one could believe their ears. Sly, now into showing off, really put her heart into singing and playing with Paw. Milt just watched, dumbfounded that his daughter could sing and play and he hadn't paid any close attention to her in a couple of years. Finally, after a mini concert Lea told everyone that the disc jockeys at the radio station had recorded this CD for Sly and had sent copies to Nashville. She explained that by Friday Toby and Ryan expected all six companies to become interested in a recording contract with Sly.

Amber spoke up, reminding everyone that Sly needed an agent. Lea told them that Toby and Ryan wanted to be Sly's agent and business manager.

Roger and Sue suggested taking a wait-and-see attitude until Milt talked with a lawyer. If and when the recording people called, they should ask questions. Paw and Mam Maw agreed with the Harts, just wait and see what happens. Everyone looked at Milt and waited until he spoke. He agreed that indeed it would be better to wait. In fact, he suggested that Mia should get in touch with one of her clients who was big in the country-music business and ask some questions. Lea, impressed as she was with Toby, agreed to put the contract signing on the back burner.

Lea asked Sly if she had anything to say since all of the fuss was over her and Paw's well-kept secret. Sly, not one to mince her words, asked, "If the recording people do call and I don't have an agent, who decides who my agent will be? Will I have any say-so or will I have to work with someone I don't know or like? If I have any say-so in this, I want Toby to handle my career and my family to handle the money."

"What about this Ryan guy, Lea? Ain't he in there with Toby?" asked Mam Maw Myers.

"I done been watching that Ryan guy. Boy, that sucker thinks he ain't nothing short of a stud muffin," said Amber.

"Yeah that's right. It's my notion that he is along for the ride and would never give up a DJ job to promote anyone else. This man is too self-centered," answered Lea, "If he couldn't handle Sly's money, I doubt he would even be interested."

"That's what I'm talking about, a good agent gets about ten per cent of an artist earnings but they wind up somehow with about a third of what the artist makes, according to the ones I know out yonder in California," said Amber. "It might be just as well to handle Sly's business in the family since all of you are business people and hire a consultant, public relations person, lawyer and whoever when you need 'em," answered Amber looking at Roger for support.

"That sounds like a winner to me, but let's just wait and see what happens in the next few days," said Paw, taking Amber's side and knowing she had been around entertainment people out in California. Roger and Milt agreed with Paw.

As the party was breaking up, Lea and Milt walked outside to see everyone off. Lea talking to Amber as they stood by her car, asked, "Amber, if all this comes to pass and Sly does make a career out of music would you help us since you have experience in this type of work?"

"Let me tell you this, up front, right now. I'm gonna be pissed off big time if I ain't in on all this from the start. I aim to see that Sly is the best-looking woman in the world, by God," answered Amber, meaning every word.

"I'm taking charge of this young'un's hair, wardrobe, and makeup when she starts her concerts. You might as well go ahead and tell Mia now so they won't be no big-ass misunderstanding later on about who's going to take care of Sly out on the road," said Amber as she hugged up Sly. Before she got into her car and left, Amber again reminded Lea, Milt, and Sly, "Get Mia straightened out about who's who on the road, Lea."

"Mama, does this mean that Aunt Mia won't have no more say-so about my clothes, hair, lipstick, nail polish, makeup and all?" asked Sly watching Amber back out of the driveway.

"Sounds like it to me, baby if you get a record contract. Amber is the best at what she does and I really like her," said Lea.

"I do too, Mom," said Sly.

During the afternoon show Ryan was rocking and knocking. Being number one in the listening area Ryan took the liberty of using his looks and influence to con young girls to his apartment to get a CD. Toby had warned him again to stop molesting the young girls before it backfired on him and got him jail time. Before the show ended he had talked three young girls into dropping by his apartment and getting a CD and probably molested as well.

Kimberly knocked on his apartment door exactly forty-seven minutes after his show was over. Ryan, in his shorts without a shirt, invited Kimberly inside. Kim, a dishwater-blonde darling, five-six, one ten pounds, brown eyes, and sporting a teenager figure was not up to her assignment. Kim's dad was assistant DA for Adams Parish. Nineteen, a college freshman, cute and petite, Kim looked fifteen. Her dad and the sheriff acting on street gossip decided to try to set Ryan up and find out exactly what was going on when he invited young girls to his apartment. Kim volunteered to call in until she got invited to his apartment.

Kim had in her purse a tape recorder she turned on before she knocked on Ryan's door. Ryan's instinct told him that something was wrong. Kim, a bad actress, couldn't walk or didn't talk like a fifteen-year-old girl. Kim was given a CD and unceremoniously shown the door. Ryan knew for sure that the law was on to him when he watched Kim get into a car parked in front of his apartment and two unmarked sheriff cars followed Kim's car as she drove away.

Toby was eating downtown. Ryan knew the locals were now on to his charade. He would not invite or let any of the young girls into his apartment for a couple of weeks and the locals would go away. It had worked before and would probably work here. Meantime he would have to satisfy himself with the sixteen-year-old girl who lived in the apartment next door with her divorced mother. She would knock on the door every morning as soon as her mom left for work with her clothes and cell phone in a gym bag to spend the morning in bed with Ryan and clean up the apartment. Hard to beat a deal like that, especially if the visitor was a cute redheaded girl with a mother who didn't really care what her daughter did as long as she stayed out of her mother's business.

When the deputy sheriff asked the redhead girl's mom if she knew that her daughter went over to Ryan's apartment every morning after she went to work, the woman's answer was "Yeah, what about it? She cleans up their apartment for them."

Sheriff Alden Malone knew that sooner or later someone would file charges against Ryan. He planned to put Ryan's ass in Angola for life when the charges were filed. Every afternoon a deputy videotaped who came and went from Ryan's apartment.

Chapter 5

Getting Sly and her mamma to their house and beelining it to her own, Mia shucked the clothes and grabbed a quick shower. White shorts, pale blue and white striped heavy-duty halter-top, sandals, and a pizza appetite, Mia headed to the local pizzeria she had sold to Sam Ebarb three years ago. Sam had spent all his adult life as a galley hand and cook working in the Gulf on offshore drilling rigs. Mia was one of the few true friends Sam had. They sat and talked a lot; Sam had never made a pass at her although the thought wallowed through his mind every time she came in to eat pizza.

Sam was from a great family that owned a fishing lodge up on the Texas side of Toledo Bend Lake. Very close to the same age, Sam was raised to know where the line in dirt was drawn and who drew it as far as Mia was concerned. She had never invited Sam to step over the line. Sam had never hit on her. Usually all men that got to know Mia hit on her sooner or later. Lately Sam had been seeing a certain, new-in-town beauty salon operator. Mia knew about the affair but never mentioned it to Sam.

Sam knew more gossip and what was happening in and around Oakwood than all four beauty parlors, the pool hall, all the coffee shops, sheriff's deputies and all the barmaids and bartenders in the parish. Mia's business thrived on good networking as it is now called, be it gossip or whatever. She had listed and sold many a property by knowing who was getting a divorce, moving away, moving in, and being there first to get the listing. Sam could gather more information in a day than all the day counters in Oakwood could in a month. He

41

loved to lay all his gossip on Mia and watch her reactions to each revelation he laid on her. He could always make her get a pen and notepad out to write down names and dates. Tonight he told Mia about Toby's asking a thousand questions about her, and also his answers. Sam told Mia that he believed that the man was infatuated with her. She simply nodded and kept listening.

Mia was paying her ticket when Toby walked in the pizzeria with Ryan. Toby walked right up to Mia and asked, "You leaving?"

"Yeah, I'm on my way to the house," answered Mia quite taken back at Toby's directness.

"If you aren't in a big hurry, hang out with us for a while. Have you eaten yet? How about a pizza?"

Turning up the charm, throwing the left hip out slightly, Mia replied, "Sure Toby, why not. Who is your friend here?" already knowing it was his friend, Ryan.

"Ryan Roberts, meet the most beautiful lady on the Gulf Coast, Mia Comeaux."

"What a pleasure to meet you, Ryan," said Mia, thinking what a hunk and noticing Ryan wore no wedding band or any jewelry on his hand. "Was listening to your show this afternoon, Ryan. Thanks for the dedication, Toby. That was sweet of both of you."

Talking to Toby and watching his eyes paint her upper body with raw, unbridled lust strangely turned up Mia's attention about three notches. Usually this strong of a come-on by a man would get nowhere with Mia. Sitting here in a pizza parlor actually enjoying a man much younger than herself peeling the clothes off her body with his eyes, she wondered if she had she become desperate. No. She reminded herself again that, by God, this is why she worked her ass off trying to stay attractive. "If I pull in a young hunk like this one then I must be doing some good." She was enjoying every minute of it. Mia's interest with the young man sitting in the booth across from her had moved from slightly to very with his impeccable manners and a voice that gave not a hint of where he was from.

Most people gathering information appear noisy or rude, usually both. Mia could glean information out of folks, especially men, like a big John Deere six-row cotton picker in a Louisiana Delta cotton field, and never seem to ask a question. In seven minutes, she knew their last names, ages, and where they worked before moving to

Oakwood. Engrossed in Toby's conversation she noticed Ryan was hardly listening and not paying any attention to her. Noting his uninterest, she started talking directly to him. Actually flirting and turning up the charm to nearly the "take me home and have your way with me" mode, she noted that Ryan did not seem even remotely interested in her. Mia carefully noted this in the back of her mind wondering if the handsome man was gay. She wasn't used to being ignored by anyone, especially a man. Period. Something was not right about Ryan. Mia decided to try to find out what his problem was.

Toby, seeing his friend getting all the attention from Mia, abruptly cut in the conversation asking if he could take her out tomorrow night since it was Saturday night.

"If you want to go dancing and drink some beer, what's wrong with right now?" teased Mia.

"Let's go," answered Toby getting his check and heading to the register to pay.

Stepping out into the late afternoon heat and humidity, Toby and Mia realized what a fine air conditioner Sam had in his place. It was quickly agreed that they would go in Mia's Yukon leaving Ryan the Corolla.

Mia drove a few miles, took a few turns, and pulled in at Bubba Ray's State Line Dance Hall and Saloon near the Texas line. Until Bubba Ray bought the club, a series of owners let the riff-raff from the whole Golden Triangle area congregate there. It got so bad that the joke was that they would issue you a gun or knife at the door if you didn't have one. Fighting inside and outside on the parking lot was commonplace as well as every other kind of misbehavior known to exist around a bar.

Bubba Ray didn't like selling used cars. He and his wife decided to reopen the dance hall after a knife fight on the parking lot where the loser almost lost his life. The High Sheriff put a bull cod lock on the front door, shutting the place down. Once big Bubba Ray took over, all of that crap stopped. Leasing the place from its owner, Bubba Ray and his wife cleaned the place up, painted, and redecorated it leaving only the galloping Clydesdales over the bar. He had his grand opening just before Thanksgiving last year.

After putting all of the riffraff's asses in the road that used to hang out there, Bubba Ray's effort began to pay off. With good bands and catering to singles, young married and middle-aged couples, the dance hall started to turn a nice profit. As crappy as it looked from the road, this was the place to take a date or wife out dancing, drink a few adult beverages, and have a great time.

Toby had no idea that his date knew almost everyone in the building. He couldn't talk to Mia or dance with her. All the men lined up for the next dance. Sitting in a booth just off the dance floor, peeling the label off a long neck, a bad case of the red-ass had set in on the jilted.

The tall cowboy who walked through the door and went directly to the bar and chug-a-lugged a draft beer got the attention of every woman in the house, including Mia. Lynn Howard was the most eligible bachelor in the Golden Triangle. Dressed in starched and ironed Wrangler Jeans, Resitol four-inch brim straw hat, tan and white western style shirt, hand-made leather belt with sterling silver buckle and conchs, and wearing a pair of plain leather Justin roper boots, Lynn dressed like a cowboy—he had horses and participated in team roping and bull dogging. Lynn could walk the walk and talk the talk.

Lynn turned and checked out the crowd on the dance floor. Single, moderately successful, and with a great personality, Lynn, an owner–operator trucker, was leased on to Paw and Milton Myers. He pulled a Utility reefer trailer with his nearly new International Eagle extended cab Pro Sleeper tractor with just about every accessory known inside and outside the unit. In truckers lingo, Lynn was known as a chicken hauler. Operating under the Myers' family authority, Lynn had made and saved some money over the years. He had never married but was a world-class womanizer. He had to be careful every time he went to party down. Lynn had elevated flirting into a fine art. It got him in lots of trouble with jealous boyfriends and husbands. Standing six-three, two-hundred eighteen pounds, he could take care of himself and the women.

"God Almighty! Talk about a good-looking woman," said Lynn to himself watching Mia cutting up on the dance floor with a young dude he didn't know. When Mia turned to face Lynn, he could not take his eyes off her. She had sold him his place outside of town and knew her well but had never thought of her as an item. Carefully scrutinizing the crowd on and off the dance floor Lynn could not for the life of himself figure out who she was with. Ordering another draught beer, Lynn took a long log-hauler sip and walked out on the dance floor as the band wound down a great version of a Willie Nelson classic, *Georgia on My Mind.* As the young man was escorting Mia across the dance floor Lynn stepped up and just took Mia away from him saying, "Bud, the next dance is promised to me," cutting the young man loose by taking Mia's arm and steering her in the opposite direction.

"Lynn, what a pleasant surprise. I didn't know you were here," said Mia, lying and hugging up Lynn, really glad to see him.

"Just dropped in for a beer or two. My truck is in the shop and I'm on my way to the house."

"How you been doing, Lynn? Haven't seen you since I sold you your place. Bet you got it looking good. Ain't been out that way in a while."

"Mia, I'm kinda disappointed in you, baby."

"Why?"

I'm sorely hurt that you ain't been out there to see me and maybe stay a day or two," said Lynn really turning up the flirting to the max.

"Lynn, you know something, Big Boy?"

"What's that darling?"

"You never got around to asking," answered Mia looking into his brown eyes, making sure that he was not joking. Lea had been matchmaking for them for years, but it had never gotten off the ground.

Lynn, two years older than Mia, was a champion high-school rodeo cowboy and still quite good to this day in team roping and bull dogging. Football and cheerleading were Mia's high school thing. She and Lynn never were on the same frequency in their high school days although, like every girl at Oakwood High, she thought he was the living end.

"You go out with them lawyers and executive type men, Mia. I always thought I'd be spinning my wheels messing with you."

"Bullshit, I've always wanted to go out with you since high school. You've acted like you didn't even like me."

Except for the twin fiddles, the house band had played George Strait's *Amarillo By Morning* damn near as good as George's *Ace In The Hole Band* could. Lynn, one of the best boot scooters around, was holding a world-class two-stepper. Matching every step, Mia was really enjoying dancing with Lynn. Spooked by Mia's directness and high-school type flirting, Lynn become extremely leery, suddenly keenly aware of everyone in the place, expecting to be invited outside at any minute by some bronckey dude and he and his buddies beat the dog crap out of him on the parking lot. Looking down into the pretty woman's eyes as the band was finishing the song, Lynn asked, "Mia, are you with somebody?"

"Yeah, I am. He picked me up at Sam's. That boy has been warting the crap out me. I finally gave in and brought him out here. He works at the radio station. I'll bet he's pissed right now."

"Why?"

"I danced with him once, and he's been over there watching every move I make. That's him in the second booth over there."

"Uh-huh."

"He's a little younger than me but he is a real nice guy, Lynn."

"I need to be getting on to the house, Mia. See you around. Come see me sometime," said Lynn ignoring her statement, turning and walking out of Bubba Ray's State Line Dance Hall and Saloon, never looking back.

Mia strolled over to the booth, slid in up next to Toby. Chatting him up in less than a minute, Toby forgot what he was mad about.

"Come on and let's dance, Toby."

"I'm glad you asked. I really enjoy dancing with a great dancer like you."

"You are full of it, Toby. Let's do this'n and spilt."

Driving back to Oakwood on the backroads, Mia asked, "Toby, is Ryan gay or what?"

Laughing and looking at Mia he replied, "No, Mia, he likes his women young, real young."

"Like nineteen or twenty?"

"No. Like twelve or thirteen," said Toby embellishing his statement somewhat, not wanting Ryan to be the topic of their conversation.

"That man a child molester or what, Toby?"

"To a certain extent I guess you could say that. He's not a predator. The only thing is that they always come to him. Ryan never goes out stalking them, never."

"Does he have a young harem beating his door down since he moved to Oakwood?"

"Yeah, but not exactly," answered Toby. "He has his eye on one particular one right now. Boy, is she a looker,"

"Who is she?"

"Can't say."

"Want to go by my place for a while?"

"No Toby, I got to work tomorrow. What do you mean by not exactly? Don't you know that kinda shit will get your ass shot off, beat to death, or put in the penitentiary for the rest of your life in this part of the country?"

"Yeah, I know that. I don't want to talk about Ryan. Let's talk about you. I want to get to know all about you," said Toby easing over toward Mia and rubbing her neck as she concentrated on driving.

Knowing she had been a tad rude and really nosy, Mia reached over and rubbed her hand up the inside of his leg from his knee all the way to his crotch and quickly removed her hand. Toby responded by doing the same to her, only he let his hand stay in the pubic area, his other hand fumbling with her halter-top.

Pulling to the shoulder of the road knowing that she could not drive and neck at the some time, Mia popped the seat belt and slid out from under the steering wheel. She turned, straddled Toby's legs, facing him, and put her lips close to Toby's. Responding with a tender kiss that grew passionately with each heartbeat, he slid her halter-top up ever so easy. When her breast fell free Toby whispered, "I've never seen anything so beautiful," as each hand caressed and rubbed the nipples now hard as nails. Bending down to kiss them, he was surprised as Mia reared back and abruptly pulled her halter down.

"I like you and what you are doing, Toby. I apologize for letting myself go like that, but we can't just park out here on the side of the highway and make out like high school kids."

Seeing the lay of his lifetime slipping away, he asked almost begging, "Can't we go to my place or yours?"

"No, we can't, Toby. I'm not going to have sex with you the first time we go out. Now get over there by that door and let me drive you home," answered Mia, sliding back under the steering wheel, now put out with herself for letting herself go for a minute with a man she hardly knew.

Mia drove directly to Toby's apartment and dumped him in the driveway with that "See you later and had a great time" smile.

Stopping for her coffee Saturday morning at the convenience store, dreading to have to work this Saturday, Mia popped the Yukon in park, pulled down the sun visor, checked her makeup, pursed her lips, made sure her lipstick was perfectly applied, and unassed the Yukon determined to make the day profitable. Dreading to show this dreadful couple yet another house, it seemed that she had shown these people a house every other weekend for the last two years. She had made up her mind that today was it, they'd have to get their minds made up or get out of her life.

Walking to the door of the store, she noticed a guy gassing up a pickup that was pulling a horse trailer at the gas pumps. The cowboy hat and pickup looked vaguely familiar. As Lynn Howard hung up the gas pump nozzle and headed for the door, Mia recognized him. She waited as he approached and smiled and said, "Good morning, cowboy,"

"Hi Mia, you working today?"

"Yeah, it's my Saturday. Whatcha' up to?'

"I'm headed to the farrier with my horse to get his shoes reset and going over to Jasper to a team roping later this afternoon."

"Going by yourself?"

"No, not if I can talk you into going with me."

"I would love to go, Lynn. What time you plan on leaving?"

"Oh, 'bout twelve-thirty or so."

"You really serious about me going with you, or just being nice, or what?"

"I'd be thrilled to death for you to go with me, Mia. Bet you never been to a team roping?"

"Never have, Lynn."

"You said you had to work today. What about that?"

"Got to show a house in Vidor at eight-thirty. After that, I'm out of there. I'll be at your house before twelve-thirty, Lynn."

48

"Gonna be waiting on you then."

"I'll be there," said Mia, hugging Lynn and looking into his dreamy brown eyes for some kind of reaction. Therein she saw what she was looking for: a macho redneck cowboy trying to act uninterested. Bingo. Mia knew those brown eyes were not lying. Desire openly radiated from them.

Meeting the couple at the office at the arranged time, Mia asked them to follow her in their car to the home in Vidor. As they walked up to the house Mia knew she would probably sell this home to the couple because the inside of house was as impressive as the neatly manicured three-acre yard. Mia had deliberately decided to show this couple a house far above the price range they had asked to be shown. She was tired of messing around with folks who couldn't make up their mind. Mia had decided that if they said anything bad about this dream home other than its price, she would ask them to find another realtor. This young chemical plant executive and his family had to put their home on the market because he was being transferred to Knoxville.

Expecting Mia, the homeowners had coffee made and were gracious hosts. If a single workmanship flaw was anywhere in the house, Mia's expert eye could not find it. Mia did not have to point out a single selling point in this expertly interior decorated and lavishly furnished home. In the breakfast room drinking coffee, Mia negotiated the price down some from the inflated asking price. Lookers became buyers on the spot. Mia quickly had both parties sign the paperwork, closing the deal and asking if they could be in her office Tuesday afternoon for formal closing. Everyone agreeing, Mia excused herself and headed to Oakwood.

As Mia approached the road to Lea's house, she saw Sly crossing the main road heading toward her house. As she crossed the road and started down the road toward her house peddling her bike, Aunt Mia pulled alongside her and stopped. "Where have you been, Sly?" asked Mia.

"Playing and singing with my friends."

"Oh, I was just wondering what you were doing over this way."

"What are your plans for later?" asked Sly.

"Oh baby, do I have big plans."

"What kind of plans, Aunt Mia?"

"I'm on my way to your house. Your Mama has to help me get dressed western for this afternoon."

"Why?"

"I'm going to a team roping with Lynn."

"You mean he's finally asked you out?"

"Yeah, I've always liked Lynn."

"Better be careful Aunt Mia. The word is that he is a handful, if you know what I mean. Mama said he is the best-looking single man around."

"Tell your Mama I know how to handle a man like Lynn."

"Sure took him a long time to get around to asking you out."

"Yeah, it did. Get on the house. We got to get out of the middle of road. A car is coming. Bye," said Mia as she drove away thinking, "My baby surely hasn't been in that damn radio station with Ryan and Toby." Turning at the next street, Mia quickly turned around and headed back to the radio station to see if the disc jockey's car was there. She saw the car that was at Sam's last afternoon sitting there big as a pimple on a teenager's cheek.

As Mia turned through the parking lot, the inside of her eyes and nose literally ignited and burned with rage.

"If that pedophile son of bitch has fooled with my baby down there, I'll have Milt and Lynn to kill him—may both of them bastards," screamed Mia as she hit the steering wheel hard enough to bruise her hand. Biting and sucking on the heel of her bruised hand Mia pulled into the Lea's driveway. She tried to calm herself before Lea saw her and started asking questions. Mia lit a cigarette and took a long drag and blew smoke on the windshield not even cracking the window. Thinking back to what was said, Sly had mentioned friends. "Surely she's not friends with Ryan and Toby. She was probably at some girlfriend's house on down the street," said Mia, answering her own thoughts.

Sly was holding the door open for Mia and had already told her mama why Aunt Mia was here. Lea, dressed in jeans and tee shirt and grinning asked, "So Lynn has finally seen the light and asked you out?"

50

"Yeah, he did. I'm going with him to a team-roping thing over in Jasper. I got to meet him at his house before twelve-thirty. I need to get dressed western, and I need your help."

"All you got to do is dress like you were going out to a country western bar to line dance and you'll be fine," said Lea.

"What about some boots."

"You must have at least three pairs of lace-up ropers. Just put on the worst looking pair and you will be fine."

"I don't have a western belt or cowboy hat."

"You need don't a western belt, Mia. Only women barrel-racers wear them to show off their prize belt buckles. I got a straw hat you can use. Sly, go get your hat and my new one and let's see which one looks the best on her."

In seconds, Sly put both hats on the kitchen bar. Lea carefully placed Sly's hat on Mia's head. It would do but was just a tad small. Lea backed up and looked carefully at Mia, then Sly. Sly shook her head indicating that her mom try the other hat on Mia. Lea then put her own hat on Mia.

Sly and her mom looked for a moment and Lea announced, "Mia this is you. It fits right and looks just right."

"Mama's right, Aunt Mia. That hat turned you into a real cowgirl," said Sly.

"Don't want to be a cowgirl. I just don't want to look out of place."

"Well, take that hat and go home and get ready before he leaves without you," said Lea picking at Mia.

Carefully dressing and putting on makeup after a quick shower, Mia pulled into Lynn's driveway at eleven fifty-five looking great. Bo, Lynn's Blue Heeler, announced her arrival running to the Yukon to meet her. For some odd reason she remembered his name. "Get back, Bo. You better get used to me being out here, big buddy."

Bo wagged his tail and led her to the steps of the trailer. Lynn opened the door and came out on the small porch built on to the side of the small doublewide trailer.

"You are really looking good, Mia. 'Bout ready to leave if you are?" he said.

"I'm with you, Lynn. I just wanted to get here a little early and not hold you up and all."

"Come on in while I finish getting my stuff together, and we'll head on over to Jasper."

Mia remembered what a mess the inside of the doublewide was when she sold this place to Lynn. Dreading to go into what she thought would be a boar's den, she was completely taken aback at the changes Lynn had made inside the doublewide. The kitchen and dining room floor was new linoleum, nice carpet in the living room and bedrooms. The walls were refinished, doors, and cabinets were all redone and finished with a polyurethane natural finish. Not a dirty dish sat on the cabinet or in the sink, every bed was made up, no clothes scattered all over The place was as spotlessly clean as a Marine barracks and smelled real good.

"My God, Lynn. You have really fixed up this place and it is so neat and clean."

"I've got it just about like I want it. I have a Mexican girl who comes over every day to feed my horses and Bo. She also cleans up after me."

"Man, would I like to hire her to keep my house nice and clean like this," said Mia.

"She probably needs the money, but she don't have a way to go."

"I could arrange transportation for her if she is interested."

"Okay, I'll ask her if she is interested."

"You do all this work yourself?"

"Naw, I had help. Dad and my buddies helped me get this place whipped in to shape. I'm 'bout ready. You?"

"Let's go," said Mia, heading out the door.

Lynn loaded two of his horses into a nearly new gooseneck Sundowner horse trailer with a small air-conditioned cubicle ahead of the horse compartment for changing clothes and showering in the front section. Complete with a bunk bed and toilet, the trailer was a cowboy's dream for rodeos and match events. Lynn had a portable generator and water tank in case no electricity and water were available. Lynn wasn't going off anywhere half-assed fixed. His '98 Chevy pickup was as clean and nice as Mia's new Yukon. With Bo in the back sitting on the toolbox, they headed for Jasper, Texas.

Mia's eyes raked Lynn up and down six or eight times as he drove out of Oakwood toward the Texas line. She wondered why this man had never married, never even serious about a woman, as far as she knew. Is something wrong with him or is he just the bachelor type? Lately Mia had been thinking maybe it was time to find the right man and start her own family. After all Sly will be leaving for college in three years. The thought of marriage always rubbed her the wrong way until lately. Maybe getting past thirty changes folk's outlook. "If and when I get married, I want this man," said Mia to herself, almost out loud.

Chapter 6

"It has to be forbidden or against the law or something. Something that good has to be forbidden, Lea. That man could have had his way with me before we got back to his house Saturday night. I wonder why most women never date Lynn but once or twice," questioned Mia, expecting Lea's answer to validate her apprehension concerning Lynn's bed-hopping.

"You saying something weird or queer may show up in Lynn on your next date, Mia?"

"If he has a flaw, I didn't find it, Lea. He was the best. A real man, the kind I like to be around.

"Are you saying he's good in bed, Mia, or what?"

"That man is great in bed, out of bed, or whatever. He's just a great guy."

"One date and you are in love with Lynn?" asked Lea.

Biting on her bottom lip and squinting her black eyes, Mia nodded affirmative. "I just really wanted to see what he was like. I spent the weekend with him, and I've got a crush on him. I know he dates lot of women and I've got lots of competition, but I think he really does like me. I'm making my move on him. I intend to marry Lynn Howard, if he don't have a split personality or something, Lea. He is the one I've been waiting on."

"Yeah, you gonna have lot of competition. Is he endowed like I heard he was?"

"You know, I had never heard that he was, but I sure found out. If he wasn't really easy at first I could not have handled him at all. After the first time, everything went great but we had to be very careful. He is so sweet and considerate, Lea. Not like most men that only worry about satisfying themselves."

Lea was driving and Mia was sitting with a cup of coffee and a cigarette, talking as they rode toward Beaumont in Lea's Suburban, not going anywhere but riding and chatting in complete privacy. This kind of talk had gone on between them since they each had started having sex with men. Lea didn't have lot of sex stories since her husband was great in bed, and Mia knew all about their sex life. Lea loved to listen to Mia rave about one of her lovers and ask questions about them. It didn't bother either one of them to ask any kind of very personal question about their sex lives. They always were honest with each other and laughed a lot about some of Mia's escapades.

Today was different. Mia had mentioned the "M" word when talking about Lynn. This was something special. Just the other day Mia mentioned having a baby before she got too old.

Talking slowed a bit and Lea said, "Mia, I got a CD here I'm going to play, and I want you to tell me who is singing." Pushing the right buttons, the intro music for the number one country song faded as the young woman began to sing.

Mia listened closely for half the record finally asking, "Who is that singing?"

"You don't know who that is singing that song? You know her."

"No, I don't know, Lea. Who is it?"

Lea smiled and said, "Now listen to this song," pushing buttons to bring up another song on the CD.

The Suburban speakers filed the truck with the music and voice of Sly's record that she and her Paw wrote and Ryan and Toby recorded it. Mia sat shaking her head. She had not heard Sly sing since she was a child. Mia finally said, "If I know her, I know a girl who's going to be rich singing. She is really great."

Tears of pride welled up Lea's beautiful hazel eyes. Her chin and voice was quivering when she quietly said, "That's Sly, Mia. That's my baby singing.

"You are bullshitting me?"

"I'll swear it is her. When we get home, I'll ask her to sing for you. She had to prove it to me and Milt. This is what I had the party for Mia. Milt and I are thinking about letting her go big-time."

"Well, are you making any plans for her?"

"No, we thought we would just let it slide for a while and see what happens."

Suddenly Mia's nostrils flared as rage literally turned her dark eyes into a ghoulish green color. She turned and screamed at Lea, "Ryan—that pedophile son of a bitch at the radio station—he made this CD, didn't he, Lea? I will kill that bastard!"

"What pedophile? What are talking about, Mia? What's this pedophile crap you talking about?" asked Lea, completely confused by Mia's tirade.

"Ryan Roberts is a pedophile, Lea. I don't want Sly within a mile of that no-good child molester. Are you hearing me, Lea? `Hello?"

"He seemed to be such a nice guy,. Mia."

"Nice guy? Listen to me, woman. That lowbred bastard is hitting on every young girl he can talk to down there at that radio station. Whatcha mean nice guy? Lea, please don't tell me this bastard has been to your house? He is a grown man that has his way with little girls. Are you hearing me, woman?"

"No. Wait a minute. Sly and I went down to the radio station to thank him for the CD. He and Toby sent copies of this CD to their contacts in Nashville."

"Did you thank him for molesting your daughter and my godchild? You keep my baby away from this child-molesting bastard, Lea. Do you hear me?"

"Wait a minute. Just how do you know Ryan is a child molester?"

"Because I went out the other night with his partner, Toby. He flat out told me that Ryan was a sicko pedophile. That is why they are here and not at some humongous radio station, Lea. How many times has she been around him alone? You really need to talk to her, Lea. Don't fuss and raise hell with her. Just find out what you can. She will be sexually active soon enough, but at fourteen with a man damn near our age, I damn sure don't think so. If I find out that no-good bastard has molested her, I will cut his tally-wacker off and shove it up his perverted ass myself," tiraded Mia.

"I don't believe Sly would let something happen as much as we preach to her about men," said Lea trying to calm Mia and reassure herself at the same time.

Not letting the issue rest for one moment, Mia countered with, "You know what?"

"What?"

Looking toward the back of the Suburban as if to make sure no one was listening, Mia turned and slowly lit another cigarette and took a long deep drag, leaving the "what" screaming for an answer. Cracking the door window and blowing the ash off her cigarette, Mia turned a said, "Do not under any circumstance let Milt or Paw find out about this, Lea. I will handle it for you. Milt and Paw will kill that man if they even suspect him of molesting her and you know it. We don't need a killing on our hands but we do need to get these two bastards out of Oakwood and in a jail somewhere."

"But we don't know for sure that Ryan has messed with Sly, Mia."

"You know damned good'n well if he's screwed four other young girls he already has hit on Sly. Shit, what's wrong with you, Lea? Some of them bastards butter up the parents just to get a chance to molest their child. No sirree, Lea, this shit gotta stop now."

"What can we do to get to help with this, Mia?"

"Don't know right off, but I'm gonna talk to Amber. She knows all kinds of people that know how to do dirt on people. We can get them run out of town."

"What if he has already messed around with my baby?" asked Lea, tuning up to start crying.

"Pull over and let me drive, Lea,"

Already crying and shaking, Mia hugged her best friend calming her somewhat as they changed places. Mia took another long drag off her cigarette and sat behind the steering wheel making no move to leave. Before she put her foot on the brake and pulled the Suburban into drive, she looked Lea straight in the eye and calmly declared, "If he did he is a dead man. He will never leave here alive. Trust me."

Lea promised to talk to Sly and find out what the story was behind the CD. When she found out something, she would let her know.

Late leaving Oakwood for work, Mia decided to show up at the office for a while, then ease out and find Amber. Most beauty salons were closed on Monday; Amber's place was no exception. Where would she find Amber on a Monday? She had to laugh to herself at the thought of that heifer laying up with Sam Ebarb, thinking nobody don't know nothing about their torrid affair.

Mia slipped away after checking on everything and leaving the girls in the office to take care of things. She knew where Amber lived but had never been to her place. Amber had rented a mobile home out in the trailer park on the east side of town. Mia didn't know which trailer but she knew what kind of car she drove. Mia just cruised the trailer park until she found Amber's car. Middle of the morning sun had already gotten a sultry day kicked off when Mia knocked on Amber's door. She knocked three times, nothing happened. Finally Mia left the porch heading toward her car, cussing herself for not calling ahead first. Suddenly Amber shouted, "I can't get no sleep out here for people beating my damn door down! Come on in here and tell me what brings you out here without calling first, Mia."

Amber stood in the threshold holding the door open for Mia as they looked each other over. Amber wore only a oversized man's tee shirt and a pair of satin men's boxer shorts showing off her great body. Mia was dressed in blue slacks, yellow blouse, and comfortable brown loafers.

"Want a cup of coffee?" Amber asked.

"Yeah, let me fix it," said Mia going to the coffeepot. "Did I wake you up?"

"Damn shore did. This is my day to lay up and not do nothing," said Amber, fixing herself a cup of coffee.

"At least you been up long enough to make coffee," said Mia.

"Naw I ain't. That thang's got a timer on it. I was fixin' to get up anyhow. So whatcha doing out here, Mia? Something's wrong, ain't it?" asked Amber, cleaning off a spot on the table to set her coffee and lighting a cigarette.

Mia pushing back dirty dishes and empty beer cans found a place for her coffee cup and fired off a cigarette herself. Taking a long drag she turned and faced the knowing eyes of Amber saying, "Yeah, Amber something's is big-time wrong."

"Want to talk about it a little bit and maybe try to figure something out? I'm pretty good at figuring stuff out. Just look at the shit I've been in and out of all my life."

"Here is the deal, Amber," said Mia, telling her the whole story about Sly and the CD and her concern that Ryan had already got to

Sly. Mia told Amber that Lea was asking the hard questions today. She told Amber that no matter what Sly told her mom, these kinds of questions almost always never get answered completely and honestly. In other words, she didn't expect Sly to be completely honest with her mom about Ryan right now.

"You think Ryan has already had sex with Sly, Mia?"

"We have no way of knowing. If he promised her a record deal in exchange for sexual favors—maybe."

Sam told me the other night that Ryan was a child molester. His waitress said he had his way with a thirteen-year-old the other day at his apartment. The younger they are, the better he likes 'em, is what Sam said. How did Sly get messed up with this sicko dickhead to start with? Don't her mama keep a good sharp eye on her?"

"Yeah, she does. She has a bike and rides it a good bit. 'Guess that was how she got away to meet this man. The truth is that I don't know yet."

"If you think Ryan has had his way with Sly, what do you all plan to do about it?" asked Amber.

"We don't want Milt or Paw to ever find out about this. If they do, Paw and Milt will kill Ryan and Toby. We don't want that."

"If we take care of this ourselves and do it right, Mia we will need at least one man to help us. Do you know a man you can trust to never, ever talk?" asked Amber, readily involving herself in her friend's problem.

"I think so. I need to do a little checking, though. Can I depend on you to help us, Amber?"

"Hell, yeah. I never could stand a child molester. Gays and lesbians never bothered me. I was around 'em all time out in California. Hell, I had a little affair with a lesbian. It wasn't to bad, but she just wasn't a man. I finally run her ass off and got me a man."

Mia stood and said, "Let me find out exactly what's gone on so far. If I have to, I'll get Sly off to ourselves and ask her point blank. I AM her godmother. See you later, maybe late this afternoon or tonight. Bye."

Mia decided to go by Lynn's place and see if he had made it home. He left very early on a short run and said he would probably be back early. She drove up in the driveway finding his big truck gone. Backing out of the driveway, she saw Lynn coming down the road.

Mia backed up so Lynn could park. She pulled back in the yard and got out to check on Lynn. He was already out of his rig when she walked up. To her surprise he grabbed her, kissed her hard on the lips, and then kissed her neck as she squirmed in his arms. Bo was barking because he was jealous of the attention his master was giving Mia. Lynn had her hand and was leading her toward the house and asking her what she was doing out this way. She told him she had business close by and dropped by to see if he had made it home yet.

"Did you miss me already?" asked Lynn.

"Yes, I really enjoyed this weekend. I hated to see it end," said Mia.

"It don't have to end," Lynn said as he held the door open for her.

Stopping just inside the door Lynn reached for her again. Mia stepped into his arms and tilted her head for more kisses. More kisses quickly led to the bedroom and clothes falling to the floor as the lovers passionately devoured each other's lust.

Later, lying on the bed holding each other, Lynn took Mia by the hand, got up and led her to the bathroom, and started the shower. Mia immediately thought, "Here is where the weird shit starts." Laying out towels Lynn got in the big shower tub combo with her. Both bathed each other and horsed around a bit.

Before Mia left, she asked Lynn if he would come over to her house later. Lynn jokingly said, "Baby, I'm thinking about moving in over there or you can move in over here.

"I'm for living with you no matter where," said Mia.

"I believe you would," answered Lynn.

"I'm serious as cancer. I like sleeping with you, big boy," said Mia rubbing her hand in his crotch and stroking his half-hard member as she licked her lips provocatively with her tongue.

Not knowing what to say, Lynn just grinned and slapped her on her butt.

Mia waved as she left to go to Lea's house. Lea had called when she and Lynn were in bed. Wondering if she had her talk with Sly, Mia headed for the Myers place hoping that no hanky panky was involved with the CD.

Mia decided to drop in at Sam's, get a fountain drink, and talk to him a minute if he had time. Dinner rush hadn't started, so Mia was lucky to get him to come over and sit a minute. Not one to mince

61

words, Mia barged right in, asking Sam what he knew about Ryan. He told her basically what Amber had said. Sam finished and waited for Mia to ask another question. She didn't. Sam knew something was troubling Mia when he asked, "Mia, let me get the girl that told me all this and see if she will talk to you about it."

Mia nodded yes, Sam went to get the girl out of the kitchen.

Sam introduced the young woman to Mia as Sandra and briefly explained to her what Mia wanted to know. Sam turned and left them in a booth. Mia asked Sandra if she knew the young girl involved. Sandra answered, "Yes'm, I know her. She is related to my boyfriend."

"Why haven't her folks had this man arrested?"

"Her daddy is dead, killed in a car wreck two years ago. Her mama is a lush. She thinks that Beth should be selling herself to make her own money."

"You are joking!" said Mia,

"I'll swear it's the truth. Beth is a sweet girl. Ryan just had his way with her and hurt her bad."

"Do you know of any more girls he's raped?"

"I've heard that he has molested three more, Miss Mia, but I can't be sure."

"Thanks a lot, Sandra," said Mia, patting her on the arm as she left the booth.

Mia sipped her coke, dug a cigarette out, and lit it. I'm going to have to stop all this smoking. If I can get these radio bastards out of my life, everything will be great.

Sam stopped by and asked if she found out what she needed. Mia told Sam that both them bastards up at that radio station needed killing. Sam assured her that he was behind her all the way.

Arriving at Lea's house, Mia dropped her sunglasses on the seat before she got out and knocked on the door. Lea answered the door before she quit knocking. "Where is Sly?" asked Mia.

"She's in her room."

"You and her had that little talk yet, Lea?"

"Yeah, we did."

"What she say about it?"

"Well, she says she called in the other day on a contest question and won. Ryan told her to come over to his apartment and he would give her the CD she had won. I was at Paw's riding my horse so she rode her bike over to his apartment and got her CD."

"Did he mess with her while she was there?"

"According to her, no more than the older boys at school do. Just popping off and trying to touch her."

"Did he touch her, Lea?"

"Yeah, he rubbed her arm and rubbed himself against her thigh before she pushed him out of the way and left."

"How did she get that CD with her songs on it?"

"She called him and went to the radio station last Saturday morning and recorded the CD. She said you saw her as she was leaving and you came over here to get my cowboy hat."

"Who was at the radio station besides him and her?"

"Toby and the lady who's the weekend DJ."

"Did he bother her at the radio station?" asked Mia.

"No, he just listened to her sing."

"You believe her?"

"I don't have a reason not to believe her. Why?"

"One of the girls who works for Sam just told me for sure he has probably raped at least four young girls. They all come to his apartment for some reason, and then he has his way with them."

"Right now, I don't trust either one of them bastards."

"Should we put the law on 'em?"

"The law ain't gonna do shit when they show up over at their place. Wonder why one of these girls' parents didn't put the law on his ass? What's going on that somebody ain't filed some charges?"

"I ain't got a clue, but I'm going to the house and try to figure something out to get this shit stopped. I'm the last one that should be saying something about sex as much as I like it. I was sixteen when I let Paul LeJune have some. It was the first time for both of us, Lea. I liked it then and I still like it. But by God, this bastard is a grown man luring these children to his apartment, and having his way with them just ain't right. See you later," said Mia, clearly as upset as Lea had ever saw her.

Still fuming as she turned into the driveway of her beautiful home she had bought a year ago, Mia was turning her hate into a vendetta toward Ryan without proof that he had molested Sly. The rambling ranch-style brick home sat on a huge lot with plenty of trees in the front and back yard. Three bedrooms, three baths, den, formal dining and living room, laundry room, sauna and hot tub bath, huge kitchen with breakfast nook, office, three-car garage, swimming pool, and all concrete driveways made this home one of the nicest in the area.

A paper mill executive built this home and lived in it three years before he was transferred to the Northwest. Mia had been the real estate agent for the executive. She knew no one could afford or would buy the home for the fair market price because the home was not close enough to Beaumont or Lake Charles. After the executive moved, the paper company assumed the note and paid the executive equity and told Mia to sell the home at some price. Mia took advantage of the situation and made them an offer.

Mia wrote the check two days later and moved in. Sue and Roger Hart, her bosses sent their people out to put everything in perfect working order.

Mia parked her Yukon, got her house key, and went to the door. On the screen door a note. It read, "Been trying to call you all weekend," signed Toby.

She laid the note on the kitchen counter and sat on a barstool at the counter and thought for a minute. She was working out a plan. The more she thought, the more frustrated she became. How could she get Ryan away from that apartment and into a car with a young girl? Who could she use to bait him into a trap? Not Sly, for sure. Who would know somebody that would even allow their daughter to be used as bait? Bad plan. What about those horrid videos of men having sex with children? Would that turn him on?

Chapter 7

The phone woke Mia two hours later. Lynn wanted to know if he could come over and bring the young Mexican girl who kept his place cleaned up for him and work out a deal with her. "Sure, Lynn. Bring her over and we will work out something. When you coming?"

"She's here now and I thought if you wasn't busy we'd ease on over there now."

"Great, bring her on over. I'm sure we can work something out."

Mia was listening for Lynn's pickup. When she heard him drive up, she went to the door. When the girl got out of the pickup, negative vibes jack-slapped Mia. Lynn introduced her as Anna. Seventeen and attractive, olive complexion, perfect teeth, beautiful jet-black hair and very petite except her breast, outstanding and standing out, looking good. Her nipples were showing through a cotton blouse. Her cutoff jeans were short enough. Her scant makeup was applied perfectly. Anna's medium short jet-black hair enclosed her oval face with high cheekbones, petite nose, and perfect sensuous lips.

Stung for a minute, Mia thought, "Damn it to hell. Has Lynn brought his young Mexican whore out here for me to work? Her negative thoughts evaporated when Anna referred to Lynn as Mr. Lynn and answered him with "sir" and "yes sir." Anna's soft voice with only a trace of Spanish accent, perfect manners, and great smile scored big with her prospective employer. Mia gave Anna and Lynn a tour of her house and backyard with the big swimming pool. Lynn whispered, "I'm ready to go back to the house and get my stuff and move in, Mia."

Anna had heard Lynn. Mia looked at Anna, who was smiling and shaking her head indicating, "Yeah, what a great idea."

"Just carry your ass, cowboy, get your stuff, and hurry back," answered Mia trying to ignore his joking around. She showed Anna the rest of her beautiful home. They decided to get Anna a bike and she would come every other day and clean up. If it was raining, the taxi would pick her up. Mia gave Anna a house key and told her that they would get her a bike now.

The bike shopping trip was short. Anna was easy to please. The bike was put in the back of Lynn's pickup and they took Anna home. Lynn said that Mia needed to know where Anna lived in case she needed her for something.

Leaving Anna at her house, Lynn drove to his doublewide, parked, and got out. Mia got out and followed him inside. He went to his closet, got a pair of starched and ironed jeans and shirt; to his dresser, got underwear out of the dresser; to the bathroom and got his shaving gear, putting his underwear in a cloth gym bag with his shaving kit and come back into the living room where Mia was standing.

"You ready to go?" asked Lynn.

"Where to?" asked Mia.

"Your house. I've got my stuff, like you said."

"You moving in?" asked Mia, not thinking he would when she told him to go get his stuff.

"Let's see how it works for a few days. You know I'm gone a lot during the week, but I'm always home on weekends. You were serious about what you said a while ago?" asked Lynn.

"You better believe it," answered Mia, not so certain about cohabitation now that Lynn had taken her up on her offer.

Lynn and Mia walked to the pickup all hugged up. Mia had taken the halter top off before they went shopping. She wished she had it on for the trip over to her house. She liked the way Lynn couldn't keep his eyes and hands off her. She didn't need the hot halter top after all. He had her hot as a pot of collards before they got a mile down the road.

When they got Lynn's stuff put up in her bedroom and bathroom, Mia went to the fridge and opened two beers. Sitting in the den, Mia, after thinking about Lynn moving in, was beside herself that she had the man she planned to marry moving in with her after only four days. She decided to open the subject of Ryan Roberts to Lynn to see if he knew anything about him she didn't know. Lynn didn't know Ryan or anything about him but was curious to know why she had asked him about the man.

Mia didn't answer Lynn's question until he asked again in a slightly different way.

Looking at Mia for a long minute, he could see tears welling up in those beautiful black eyes. He hugged her up and tenderly nuzzled her neck, whispering, "What's wrong, baby? What has this man done to you? Tell me what's wrong, baby."

Tears rolling down her face, Mia sobbed, "Nothing to me, Lynn. He has done nothing to me. It's Sly I'm worried about. That man is a child molester. I think he has had his way with Sly."

Lynn came up off the sofa like he had been shot in the ass with hot pork skins. "How do you know this, Mia? This is a serious accusation you're laying on this ole boy."

Mia patted the sofa and said softly, "Sit down, Lynn and let me tell you the whole story." When she finished, Lynn was up pacing the floor and asking her to repeat some of the stuff she had told him.

Finally, Lynn sat beside Mia when he finished asking questions. Lynn asked again, "Milt does not know about this?"

"No, Lea and I decided not to tell him or Paw."

"Why not? They're gonna find out anyhow, Mia. Somebody's going to tell them or Mr. Roger, and then the fat will be in the fire. You and Lea are not going to involve the law in this, I assume?" Lynn asked.

"No, if we did, all they would do is ask Sly endless questions, drooling over the answers and try to make her out as a slut."

"Whatcha gonna do then, baby?"

"We don't have that figured out exactly, yet."

"You and Lea, ah, are fixing to do some dirt to this Ryan guy, Mia?"

"Yeah, we are. Big-time dirt."

"Y'all are fixing to get yo ass in a real jam if you ain't real slick bout dis, darling."

Teary-eyed and distraught, Mia looked at Lynn. Her beautiful lips were trembling. The recollection of how her low-life stepfather constantly fondled and molested her from the time she was ten years old until his accident. Mia's mom ignored her pleas to make him stop messing with her. She was afraid her abusive husband would leave her. Just days before Mia's fifteenth birthday news of her stepfather's near fatal injury in an oil field accident sentencing him to a nursing home for the rest of his life was the best news Mia had ever received. "Why couldn't something like that happen to that perverted Ryan," she asked herself. "Would serve him right."

"Why can't we just put him in that big trailer of yours and just haul his no-good ass off somewhere and forget about that bastard, or something like that?" asked Mia, wiping her teary eyes.

"You mean get him in my reefer trailer and turn the unit to freezing and haul his sorry ass off somewhere and dump him?"

Mia slid up to Lynn, softy saying, "It didn't bother him not one bit to fool Sly into coming over to his apartment and then take my baby's virginity away, Lynn. He will pay for having his way with her, one way or the other."

"Are you sure he has had his way with Sly or are you just assuming that he did?" asked Lynn.

"Yes, I am sure. If you were in Sly's place, would you tell the truth, especially if he offered to get you a big recording contract? He's has had his way with her," whined Mia.

"You want me to help you make something happen to him?"

Biting on his ear, kissing his neck, and rubbing his butt with one hand as she held him close with the other hand, she finally kissed him and stuck her tongue deep into his mouth. As she gently broke off the kiss, Mia cooed into his ear, "It's nice to have a real man around the house, Lynn." Both knew the pact was sealed without another word being said.

"It will be dark in a little bit, Lynn. Do you want to go for a swim?"

"I didn't bring my bathing suit."

"You don't need one," said Mia as she jumped up and headed for the swimming pool. "I usually turn out all the lights and go skinny-dipping."

Lynn woke early the next morning. His stirring around getting ready to go to work woke Mia. She got up and asked if she could

68

make him breakfast. Lynn wasn't a breakfast person and told Mia to go back to bed and that he would see her in a day or two. Kissing her passionately before he told her bye, Lynn hit the road to his house to get his big truck and head up to Natchitoches to pick up a load of chickens. His destination was Amarillo, Texas, and he couldn't possibly make back until Wednesday afternoon. Lynn promised to think about how to help her and Lea.

Today when Mia got dressed for work, Anna had made her some coffee. She sat and talked small talk with Anna before she went to work. Anna told her she was a senior in high school. When school started, she would come in the afternoons and weekends. She had no boyfriend right now and had to slip around to date. Her daddy wouldn't allow gringo boys to come to their home. Anna asked Mia who cut her hair, indicating she would like her own cut like that. Mia told Anna she would get her an appointment with Amber and take her down there one afternoon this week.

By habit, Mia pulled into the convenience store on her way to work. She had to have that styrofoam cup filled with coffee, and her cigarette, as she drove to work sorting out the day's activities. Lately her mind was not on selling real estate. She had her man now living with her part time for a positive, but the Ryan and Sly thing overshadowed every thing else in her life. When Lynn got back maybe he would have a plan. Her cell phone rang, mercifully pulling her thoughts away to more pleasant things. It was Lea wanting her to drop by her house after work. Quickly flipping her appointment book to today, she was free. No property to show this afternoon unless something cropped up, she told Lea.

Milt was setting up lawn sprinklers to water the lawn as Mia drove up after an easy day at the office. Lea opened the door as she walked up asking if she wanted a beer or iced tea. A glass of iced tea hit the spot for Mia. Milt came in and sat down. Lea brought him a beer without being asked. Milt took a swallow and looked at Mia, saying, "Mia, tell me everything you know about Ryan Roberts."

Surprised for a moment, Mia looked at Lea for a hint. Lea spoke up, "He knows about Ryan. He was told today after he played Sly's record for the guys at the shop this morning. Mia, one the men in the logging crew told him about Ryan,"

69

Mia, sitting in a rattan chair, hooked one leg under the other, took a sip of iced tea, got a cigarette out taking her own good time, finally lit it and said, "What I know is that he is a pedophile, Milt. We know he tried to have his way with Sly, but she says she brushed him off. We don't know for sure. He did have his way with at least four young girls, possibly more. That's all I know."

"Tricking them to come to his apartment with the promise of giving them some CD's is what I was told," said Milt.

"That's what I was told," answered Mia.

"Sly said she just brushed him off; no real harm was done," said Lea, watching Milt's every gesture knowing he was probably going ballistic any moment. She was praying that Milt didn't go off on Mia and her for keeping Ryan's sexual advances toward their daughter from him. Lea knew they were wrong for even attempting to keep her husband in the dark about Ryan's advances toward Sly. She knew that reasoning with him in that frame of mind was out of the question.

Surprisingly calm, Milt leaned toward Lea and Mia saying, "The question is now why I wasn't told about this as soon as you two found out and suspected something might not be right. Thank God Daddy wasn't out there to hear about this, but he's gonna find out about it and so is Mr. Roger. They will be pissed off big-time because they as well as myself were out of the loop. It is my right to know that stuff like this is going on and not be kept me in the dark. It's a man's job to right this wrong, damn it. Even if Sly did put him in his place, that bastard has hit on Sly and them other little girls. Whether he had his way with them or not, he needs to be dealt with. You women don't know how to handle stuff like this like a man does."

Milt continued, "I know both of you meant well, but I'm going to take care of this situation myself. First off, I'm gonna tell Daddy and Mr. Roger and let the shit go ahead and hit the fan," said Milt standing up. Lea stood and hugged her husband. Milt motioned to Mia come close as he hugged his wife. Mia got up, and soon all three were hugging. This was the first time Milt had ever hugged Mia. Milt was finally accepting her as family. Both women were now softly crying. Tears were welling in Milt's eyes as held them tightly.

"Milt, I've told Lynn all about this and we were going to take care of Ryan. Lea and I just don't want to see you, Paw, and Mr. Roger get in trouble. We didn't exactly call ourselves hiding something. We are

70

trying to protect the whole family here. I'm part of this family too," said Mia softly with big crocodile tears rolling down her cheeks. "You not going to the sheriff with this, are you, Milt?" asked Mia.

"Not till I talk to Daddy and Mr. Roger, Mia. I'm not doing a thing on my own yet," answered Milt.

"If Lynn comes up with a good plan, would you go along with it if it gets rid of Ryan and makes him suffer for what he's done?" asked Mia.

"I might listen, but like I said, I'm gonna talk to Daddy and Mr. Roger first. Daddy is gonna want to shoot that bastard. You know that, don't you?" said Milt.

"Yeah, I know that and I understand. But is there any way you can wait and talk to Lynn before you tell Paw and Mr. Rogers, Milt?" asked Mia. "Lynn will be home tomorrow afternoon."

Rubbing his chin and looking out the window at nothing Milt thought a minute before answering, "No later than tomorrow evening."

"I'm going to the house and call him and tell to come on home quick as he can."

"From what Lea tells me, Lynn is probably gonna tear that old truck up trying to get back to the house. Y'all done jumped the broom over there, I hear," said Milt changing the tempo and picking at Mia.

Joking back at Milt, Mia replied, "I gotta get him house broke and all, Milt."

"I'm proud for both of you. Y'all should have been together all along. I know both of you will be happy. Lea said y'all are talking that talk."

"If I can get him to walk that walk, I'll be happy. I'm bout ready to start my own little family, Milt."

"Lea and me will be there for both of you. Tell him to get that ass on to the house. We got problems to handle."

"I'll tell him. Bye," said Mia walking out to her Yukon now feeling somewhat better after talking to Milt.

Watching Mia back out of the driveway Lea hugged her husband up and thanked him for not crawling all over Mia for meddling in their business. "She is as she said a part of our family, Milt. She loves Sly as much as we do. She refers to Sly as her baby." Suddenly Lea turned her husband loose and popped down in the rattan chair Mia was sitting in. She started to cry uncontrollably. Milt, flabbergasted, tried to console her. Finally he got her to tell him what the matter was.

"I only want to punish Ryan and make him go away, Milt," said Lea.

"So what, ain't that what we all got on our mind?"

"No," said Lea.

"What is it then?"

"Mia wants Ryan punished, and then maybe killed outside of the law."

"Bullshit, I don't know 'bout that. Maybe we ought to go ahead and call Daddy and Mr. Roger and get the law involved before somebody gets in some real trouble. But I'm gonna tell you this right now, Lea. Before God as my witness, if that man laid a hand on my baby he is a dead man. I'm gonna be on Mia's side then, Lea," said Milt getting all torqued up.

"You told Mia you would wait on Lynn, Milt."

"Only till late tomorrow evening. Lynn better get that ass on to the house and get in touch with me as soon as he gets home. If he don't I'll take care of this myself," said Milt.

Allen Jackson was asking everyone, *WHERE WERE YOU WHEN THE WORLD STOPPED TURNING* on the radio. Listening to the superb stereo system in his big rig, Lynn thought for a second exactly where he was almost a year ago. Since then, the President had made it hazardous to be in the terrorist business anywhere on the planet. His popularity was off the charts from the way he and his staff were handling world terrorism. Lynn, as well as almost every single trucker in the United States, was proud of his president and proud to be an American.

Lynn's thought drifted to Mia's problem and then to Mia herself. In less than a week he had become involved with the best-looking, sexiest, most successful woman in the Golden Triangle and was living with her in her house. Lynn was keenly aware that Mia's income was more than twice his was. He didn't know for sure, but according to Mr. Roger, her income selling real estate far exceeded what most doctors and lawyers earned. She was one of the best in the business, according to Mr. Roger. Mia's image walked through his mind; thinking of her controlled his mind. He had talked to her and she briefly told him of her talk with Milt. She asked that he hurry on to the house for two reasons. Watching the sun come up, Lynn was rolling down US 287 out of the Panhandle at a high rate of fuel consumption hammer down, a bit faster than the legal speed limit. The blue daybreak ground haze, overlaid with West Texas dry air, promised that it would be over a hundred on the thermometer later. Big truck tires gnawing the hot asphalt sang the going-home-empty blues as the big rig rolled out of the high plains down to the Gulf Coast.

Making good time up to Amarillo and the fact that the cold storage plant unloaded him as soon as he arrived, Lynn was ahead of schedule by at least seven hours. He had taken a good nap last night and felt fine as he pushed his big rig hard for the yard.

Lynn worried that Milt had found out so soon after Mia told him. Lynn knew what a hothead Milt could be if provoked. He knew that Milt would be honor bound to publicly whip Ryan's ass like a yard dog. Paw and Mr. Roger would see that Ryan and Toby lost their jobs and the sheriff would run both radio men's asses off, really far off, like to Alaska or somewhere.

The troubling thought was Mia. She wanted to punish Ryan and do away with him. That thought troubled Lynn to no end. Mia was upset about Ryan, but if Sly did in fact brush the man off, no real harm was done, as for as Lynn could see. Women do look at stuff like this altogether differently than men do, conceded Lynn to himself. "I'll do what Mia wants to do. I ain't 'bout to mess up the best thing that has ever happened to me," confessed Lynn aloud into the west Texas wind.

Thinking about what Mia said about getting rid of Ryan, Lynn had thought long and hard about it on the way up to Amarillo. He always came back to what she had said knowing that she didn't exactly mean it. Putting Ryan in the reefer trailer and turning it down low as it would go, thirty-two below, should get the job done.

How would they get the man isolated so he could be put in the reefer trailer? Gonna need some bait to get him away from his place to get him and not get caught. "Wonder if Anna would help me get him out to my place or somewhere else. I could hide and get him out there. Anna probably would help me if I asked her. Hell, her crazy-ass mama thinks I'm sleeping with her anyhow. I'll ask her if she will help me out with Ryan. Maybe I could put him in there, chill his ass down real good, and then let him go. Mia would never know the difference. That's what I'll do. I'll put that bastard in ole Norris Castro's trailer. Don't like him anyway and if he gets caught with the man in his trailer, so what? Hell, I slept with his ole lady after she left him and she told him about it. She wasn't good in bed. That bitch stayed drunk too much to enjoy a good time in bed. He's tried to screw me over a couple times and all. I'll just fix his wagon along with the DJ. Daddy calls it killing two birds with one rock," said Lynn to himself, now pleased with his plan. He knew that Mia would like it if Anna would go along with it.

Lynn saw Anna's new bike leaned up against the back porch when he pulled in from Amarillo. He decided talk to her right now before she went home. Sitting on the couch folding Lynn's clothes, Anna had the TV on, watching a movie. Lynn came in and sat down next to her on the couch. "How are you and Mia getting along, Anna?" asked Lynn.

"Just great, Mr. Lynn. Miss Mia is taking me to the hair stylist that she uses to get my hair cut this week. I love working for her, but I like working for you, too," said Anna.

"Man, this is one good-looking girl. If she wasn't so young I'd hit on her myself," thought Lynn to himself. "Anna, I have a question to ask you. Really it's a big favor to me and Mia. If you don't want to help us there will be no hard feelings, but I have to ask, okay?" said Lynn watching her reaction. Seeing a positive look in her soft, dark-brown eyes, Lynn asked, "Do you know Ryan Roberts, the DJ on the radio up town?"

"No, but I listen to him a good bit, Mr. Lynn," answered Anna, her brow now furrowed.

"Have you heard any bad talk about this man?"

"Well my cousin told me, Mr. Lynn that . . . ," stammered Anna looking down and shaking her head side to side, indicating something she had rather not talk about.

"Your cousin told you what, Anna?" asked Lynn louder than he meant to. "It is very important that I know about Ryan Roberts, Anna. Please tell me what you know and heard."

74

"Well, Mr. Lynn, my cousin said Ryan had his way with a fourteen-year-old girl who lives next to her. He tricked her into going to his apartment for a free CD then had his way with her. She was a virgin, Mr. Lynn. My cousin said he was brutal with her then laughed at her and threw her out. My aunt helped her stop bleeding. Her mama wasn't home, and she was afraid to tell her mama when she came home late that night," said Anna, looking at Lynn, anxious to know what this story had to do with her.

"Why didn't your aunt call the law?" asked Lynn now wondering if someone might be putting a belly stretching on the truth.

"The girl begged my aunt not to call the law. She said she would be in more trouble than she was already. Her trashy mama would beat her half to death."

"Will you help me and Mia catch Ryan so we can stop him from hurting any more young girls?"

"How can I help, Mr. Lynn?"

"I want to get you fixed up to look younger than you are and attract his attention."

"I will be the bait for your trap?"

"Exactly. Me and Milt Myers will be close by at all times till we get him out here or somewhere isolated."

"Then what are you and Mr. Milt going to do to this bad gringo?"

"Something to make him never want a young girl again."

"My mama says most all men like good-looking young girls. Makes then feel more mannish."

Forty-five minutes later Lynn showed up at Mia's house just as she pulled in from work herself. She jumped out and hugged and kissed Lynn. As they went inside Mia noticed he had just bathed. Mia asked, "Lynn, why didn't you wait and bathe with me?"

"I was too funky to wait, baby. I got home before you anyhow."

"You don't have a key to the house, do you?" asked Mia, "I had you locked out. I'm sorry, I'll get you a key today."

"I got us a plan figured out about Ryan that we can start on tonight," said Lynn getting a beer out of the fridge, offering one to Mia.

"Tell me about it before we tell Milt and Lea," said Mia shaking her head indicating that she would pass on the beer.

Telling Mia the whole plan took less than ten minutes. "You mean Anna is willing to act as bait for us?" asked Mia.

"Yeah, she likes you and me a lot, I guess."

"Where is Anna?"

"Over at my place cleaning. Why?"

"You go get her while I jump in the shower, and we will take her to Amber's and get her fixed up to catch our man."

"What about clothes?"

"I got lots of stuff that will fit her. She is almost my size."

"Great, I'll be back with her in a few minutes, baby," said Lynn.

She called Amber before she took a shower. Amber agreed to make Anna up. She told Mia she had seen her yesterday riding her new bike. Amber acknowledged that Anna would make an excellent choice for bait. Mia was ready when Lynn and Anna got back.

Mia drove her Yukon with Lynn and Anna to Amber's shop. Arriving at Amber's beauty salon, Mia, Lynn and Anna went in to see what Amber had to say about Anna. Lea came in just as Amber told Anna to stand in front of the full-length mirror behind her chair. Mia had called Lea after she talked to Amber. Lea looked at Anna then at Mia and Lynn. "Where did you find such a pretty girl to help us, Lynn?" asked Lea.

"Anna works for me and Mia. I asked her to help us catch Ryan," answered Lynn. "We need to get him off the street."

"She is certainly pretty enough to get the job done. She has natural beauty just like Sly," said Amber to no one in particular, holding Anna's head, moving it in several positions, and turning her to one profile then the opposite while studying Anna's profile in the mirror. "If we gonna make her look much younger you are going to have to get her a sports bra. Anna has way too much bosom for a fourteen-year-old nymphet. I'm working backwards here," said Amber looking at Mia. "We are trying to catch us a stud muffin, ain't we?"

"Yes, we are. Why the sports bra? I thought bigger was better," asked Mia.

"Not in this case. I usually make the young girls look older and make the older girls look younger," said Amber still looking at Anna from every angle.

"That a problem?" asked Lea.

"Hell no. I used to do this shit all time when I worked out yonder in Hollywood. Anna will look like a fourteen-year-old when I get through with her. These boobs sticking out here like this don't make Anna look like a fourteen-year-old virgin," said Amber getting down to business.

"I got a sports bra she can have. I use them when I ride my horse," said Lea.

"Good deal, Lea, but will it hold these? This girl is loaded down with boobs," giggled Amber.

"So am I," said Lea, putting her hand to her mouth and blushing, realizing Lynn was standing beside her.

"I ain't missed either one of you," said Lynn laughing, "I doubt anyone else has either. How 'bout it, Amber?" said Lynn. Amber smiled. She knew that she was definitely included in his observations.

Mia playfully elbowed Lynn in the ribs, saying, "Oh he damn sure can't keep them eyes in that head. He's gotta be checking out at every good-looking female, big boobs or not."

"Gimmie 'bout an hour or so and I'll have her fixed up," said Amber, biting her lip to keep from laughing and trying to ignore Lynn's comment in front of Mia and Lea.

"We'll be back after her then," said Mia. "I tell you what, Amber. Why don't you drop her off at my house on the way home? You need to help us get her dressed anyhow and help her get her makeup on just right."

"I can do that," said Amber. "I'm going down to Sam's with y'all to see if the stud muffin takes the bait."

"Amber, you or Mia are going to have to get Norris down to his truck later on."

"Norris has his rig down at the fuel stop. I'll go by there, crank his reefer unit, and turn the thermostat down. If he has his trailer doors padlocked, I'll see if we can open the lock. Might have to use bolt cutters on his padlock."

"I might have dated Norris if he would get that drunk-ass ex-wife off his mind. I can't for the life of me understand what that man sees in that woman," said Amber.

"Neither can I. He has talked to me several times but never asked me out. I sold his brother in law a house after Norris called me and put me on the deal. I can handle Norris," said Mia.

"Naw, that ain't gonna work, Mia. Let Amber or Lea do it. Norris knows by now that you and me are together, and he would be suspicious as hell. Not that he wouldn't try to mess us up, but Norris would be watching his back too close, if you know what I mean," said Lynn.

"Why are Norris and you at war?" asked Lea. "Besides that, I don't run around on Milt and everybody knows that."

"I dated his wife once after the divorce. She told him she slept with me, and he never got over it. We know you don't mess around, but you may have to make him think you are starting," said Lynn

"Milt is damn sure not going to let me do this. You know how he is about me, Lynn," said Lea.

"I agreed to help you and Mia. If you want this man done away with, fine; if not, call the sheriff, Lea," said Lynn walking out of the beauty parlor to Mia's Yukon. No traffic on the streets, too hot and humid. Lynn stood on the parking lot behind the beauty parlor waiting on Mia stung to the core at Lea's remark.

Hearing footsteps Lynn turned thinking Mia was coming. To his surprise Lea walked right to Lynn and hugged him up tight, cheek-to-cheek, "Those boobs are real," thought Lynn, hugging Lea back. Lea cupped his face in her trembling hands. Hazel eyes flecked with light aqua spots looked deep into his own. Her lips quivering. Her voice was barely audible as she said, "Lynn, I'm so sorry. I know you want to help, and I've been such a prude. Please accept my apology. I will do whatever you want me to. I will tell Milt instead of asking this time. Okay?"

Looking into her eyes Lynn could see two things. One was the desire for him to forgive her and help. The other was something he could sense as a man as she still held his face cupped in her hands. She looked him straight in the eye. Lynn realized at that moment that she would do whatever he wanted her to do. Anything. Her hands released his face. Lea's desire to kiss Lynn was gnawing and shaming her at the same time. She couldn't imagine what had come over her. This was Mia's man and soon to be fiancé that she wanted to passionately kiss. She felt deeply repentant of her inclination to move on Lynn knowing Mia had never ever showed any inclination to even flirt with Milt after all these years. Mortified knowing that Lynn had read her thoughts and was interested, Lea looked at Lynn, then hung her head.

Lynn looked around to see if anyone was near and said softly, "Lea, I will help you every way I can. Don't be such a prude, though. You hear me?"

"Yeah, I hear you, Lynn. You think I'm a prude?"

"No, not at all. I think you are one great woman, said Lynn adding, "If Milt and I weren't such great friends, who knows? I would probably be your husband. Remember, I dated you before Milt."

"I remember it well, Lynn. You ain't still mad at me about that, are you?"

"No, Lea. We will use Amber if we can, but we are going to need you to help us pull this little trick off," said Lynn hugging her.

Lynn released her and for a moment, she looked deep into his eyes again. The hazel eyes wantonly communicated that silent infidelity message all men like Lynn watch for. Lea turned and went back inside.

"Got your ass put in place real quick, huh, Lea?" teased Amber.

"Damned shore did. I didn't know he was as hair-triggered as Milt. Gonna have to handle that man very carefully, Mia. I guess I was being prudish about Norris. Hell, I might get him off and seduce him," joked Lea.

"Mia, not to change the subject, but we gotta talk about these split-leg cut-off jeans Anna has on if we gonna make her look like a virgin fourteen-year-old teenager. Little too short maybe for a fourteen-year-old young'un to have on uptown?" asked Amber.

"Shit, I don't know. Sly couldn't ever own a pair like that. But, Anna has had boyfriends and sex. She can wear what she likes. Who are we to tell this girl what to wear?" asked Mia.

"Sly couldn't go up town with those split leg cut-offs on, but if it suits Anna I'm all for it," said Lea.

"I will wear what you want me to wear, Miss Mia. I just like for men to notice me. I want to help you and Mr. Lynn get Ryan Roberts," said Anna, looking at Mia for approval.

"Look, Anna, I am not trying to put you down for the way you dress, but this Ryan guy probably likes the innocent-looking type that's just getting their feet wet so to speak, sexually," said Amber.

"But fourteen ain't too young to be doing a little shopping around and testing the water far as I'm concerned."

"Good God, Amber, don't tell me you were having sex at fourteen?" asked Lea.

"Damned right I was. Not much cause Daddy and Mama watched us too close. Billy Jack Rhymes used to slip up and peck on my window after bedtime, and I would slip out and be with him. He was lot older than me but he was good to me. His big ole lard ass wife never found out, and neither did my daddy. Somehow I always believed Mama and my sisters knew I was slipping out but never told my daddy," said Amber.

"Amber is probably right about this innocent look, girls. Let's get some regular shorts or cut-offs on, a sports bra with a blouse. A tee shirt will expose what we are trying to cover up. If this won't attract him then we will stick those boobs on out there and put her in the sexiest shirt we can find. What ya'll think?" asked Mia turning the subject off Amber's past sexual stories that any other time every woman in the beauty parlor would have loved to hear.

"That'll work for me," said Amber. Whatcha think, Lea?"

"Sure, that's fine. Are you comfortable with this, Anna?" asked Lea.

"Yes ma'am, that's fine with me" said Anna.

Arriving about an hour later at Mia's house, Amber along with Anna went inside to dress for the trip to Sam's. Inside in Mia's spare bedroom Mia had shorts, shirts, panties, tennis shoes, anklet socks, and bras spread out on the bed, and in the chair by the bed as well as on the dresser. Lea had gone home and returned with two different styles of sports bra. Waiting for Anna to disrobe, Amber finally said, "Anna, do you want us to leave so you can dress. Are you shy about changing in front of us?"

"No ma'am, I was waiting to be told what to do and what to try on. I don't mind you seeing me in my underwear, Miss Amber. I'm proud of my body," said Anna.

When Anna disrobed, they could not take their eyes off her exquisite young body. She dressed according to what Mia handed her to put on. She soon looked the part of a fourteen-year-old nymph. Amber took her into the bathroom and helped her with her make up and combed her hair again. Putting the finishing touch on her makeup and standing back admiring her work Amber had definitely crafted stud muffin bait.

Lynn could not believe the radical change in Anna's looks. She could pass the fourteen test easily. Lynn had unlocked Norris's trailer. He and Norris had the same trailer locks since both had their rigs were leased on to Milt's and Lea's trucking company, pulling company-owned reefer trailers.

It was nearing five-thirty and time to call Sam's to find out if the radio guys had shown up yet. Sam said no, but they would be there shortly. They had ordered a pizza to eat in.

Lynn had put Anna's bike in his pickup and told everyone he would bring Anna to the back street and let her ride up to Sam's. He instructed Anna not to speak to Mia, Lea, Amber, Milt, or him when she went inside. She was to order a drink and sip on it until Ryan noticed her. If Ryan wanted to meet with her, she would go to his place (Lynn's) and call him to come over. Lynn gave her a ten-dollar bill before she got in his truck to go uptown.

The late August afternoon was hot and muggy. Not much traffic moving, staying cool was the deal. Norris was finally located in a bar out on the Beaumont highway, shooting pool. It would be easy enough for Amber to ease in there and get him to take her down to his truck and get into the sleeper with him. He wouldn't even be out a motel room bill. Mia and Lynn with Lea, Milt, and Amber showed up just after Anna arrived. Sam wasn't told what was going down. Lynn and Milt agreed that he didn't need to know. Both men knew he talked too much.

The whole party sat at a big round table and ordered beer. Sam pestered the hell out of them about eating. Amber told him they wanted to drink a beer or two before they ordered something. Anna was looking good sitting over there, sipping her fountain drink. Two black men come in and made an order to go. The phone was steadily ringing. Folks refusing to cook supper in a hot kitchen were ordering pizzas to go. Sam's was busy this afternoon.

Arriving just as the cook set their order on the counter, Ryan and Toby entered and looked around before they sat in a booth on the west wall in plain sight of everyone. Ryan's eyes found Anna forthwith. On the east side of the room, the round table afforded all sitting there an unobstructed view of the radio guys. After being served, Ryan again checked out the room, ascertaining that probably Anna was alone and riding the bike parked outside.

As if on cue, Anna got up and sauntered over to the jukebox near Ryan and Toby's booth and studied the huge selection. She looked over at Ryan and smiled her best smile and took a dollar and put it in the jukebox and pushed a selection. Watching the jukebox go through its ordeal, her first song began to play. Getting in to the rhythm of the country song playing, she punched out her other two songs and started back to her table.

Ryan waved her to come over. Anna went over to their booth and stood there a minute, then sat down by Ryan. Mia could see her laughing and talking to both men as they eat their pizza. Anna sipped her drink and smiled. Ryan was coming on to her big time. Everyone at the round table could tell. "Shit. I didn't know this would go this easy," said Mia under her breath.

"We ain't got him out of here and away from his buddy yet," said Lynn adding, "It's damn shore fixing to happen, though."

A slight problem was fast developing. Ryan was already rubbing Anna's leg out of sight of everyone. Anna was liking what he was doing and thought he was a great-looking man. She looked over toward the round table and Lynn jerked his head toward the door indicating that it was show time. Anna quickly removed Ryan's hand and said, "It is time for me to go. Wish I could stay longer but I can't."

"Would you like to have that album that song is on you just played, Anna?" asked Ryan.

"Yes, I sure would, Ryan," answered Anna.

"Come over to my apartment and I'll give you one. The record companies send them to me all the time to give away. I'd love for a pretty girl like you to have it," said Ryan pouring it on like syrup.

"I can't go to your place. I'm house watching for a man and he is going to call shortly checking in on me. You could come over there later and bring it to me? I would very much like to have it," Anna said, slowly licking her lips to moisten them. "You want the phone number, Ryan?" she asked.

"Sure, why not? I'll bring the CD over and visit a while."

"I'd really like that. You can stay as long as you like. I'm just going to watch TV," said Anna.

"Here is my cell-phone number. Call when you get there and are ready for me to drop by," said Ryan handing her a paper napkin he had quickly wrote a number on.

"See you later," said Anna, getting up and leaving. She went outside and got on her bike and started to Lynn's place. Ryan and Toby didn't notice the folks at the round table leave as soon as Anna left. Lynn and Mia caught up with Anna before she got home. Lynn stopped and loaded the bike into the back of his pickup. Anna jumped in beside Mia.

"What's the deal, Anna?" asked Lynn.

"He can't come tonight; he's got other plans. He did give me his telephone number and told me to call tomorrow after six," lied Anna.

"I wish to hell he would have come tonight," said Lynn "We had it all set up to get his ass."

"I will call him later. He seemed very interested in me. He might come out later on," said Anna. "Will you be over at Miss Mia's if he decides to come over?"

"Yes, he will definitely be at my house, Anna," said Mia, giggling and rubbing Lynn's leg.

"I will call then if he comes," said Anna waiting for Lynn to take her bike out of the pickup.

Anna quickly fed and watered the horses and Bo. She ran into the house and tore her clothes off and showered. She had taken a packet of that good-smelling body lotion Miss Mia had in a bowl on her bathroom vanity. She smelled her hands and the scent was just right as she rubbed her body down with it. Changing into a pair of cut-offs with the legs slit almost up to the waistband, she found one of her sexiest halters she had in the bedroom dresser and put it on. Anna picked up the phone and dialed.

Chapter 8

Amber found Norris at a local watering hole appropriately named Hideaway Lounge. Nearly a quarter of a mile off the Beaumont highway and four miles out of town, this bar sported three pool tables, three video poker machines, a loud jukebox, small dance floor, gravel and shell parking lot, and a reputation as a place to pick up a date. Lots of women and men on the prowl came here to check the crowd for a one-night stand. Loggers, construction workers, oilfield hands, truckers, loafers, and a few pool sharks were the usual clientele of this establishment. Most of the women that did patronize this establishment regularly were as rough and rowdy as the men customers. Occasionally a working girl would wander in, turn a few tricks, and leave before the law showed up. The long and short story of this place is that The Hideaway Lounge is about as redneck and Cajun honky-tonk as you could find. You would never be approached by an insurance salesman or a gay person in the Hideaway.

Naturally, when Amber eased into the Hideaway that late afternoon, every eye in the house scanned her with admiration overlapping into skepticism. Was she here to start trouble or take somebody's man or what? Amber was dressed much too nicely not to attract all the men's attention. Red and white western cut shirt showing Grand Canyon cleavage, painted-on jeans, perfect short hairstyle, and lace-up roper boots were supposed to attract attention. They did. The owner had known Amber for years; they'd been classmates in high school. She hugged his neck and sat down on a barstool close to the pool table that Norris was playing on.

Norris was better than the average barroom pool player but not in the big money, pool-shark league. Amber watched a two games of eight ball and got up and put her money on the pool table rail, indicating that she would play a winner after another player. Norris was tearing the competition's heart out. He was shooting better than usual and crowing about it to anyone who would listen. Norris never gave the young oilfield roustabout shooting ahead of Amber a shot. He took the roustabout's money and told him to go get some practice and come back.

It was Amber's turn now to play Norris. He began to badger her right off the bat. Amber picked her cue stick carefully while waiting for Norris to break the balls and carefully chalked her cue tip. Norris made a hard break, but no balls fell into the pockets.

Amber carefully scrutinized his leave before she made her move. Her aim was perfect, her leaves professional. Norris stood at the bar watching as his ass was waxed to the nth degree. Amber moved in to take control of his humiliation, indicating that she was much more interested in him than in shooting pool. Norris, not stupid as Lynn thought, saving face and knowing a good thing when it came his way, walked over to the cue rack, hung up his stick, and sat beside Amber. She forfeited her winning game.

Silent sighs of relief came from the other women in the Hideaway. Most of the men were now envious of Norris. Sexual and sensuous Amber took Norris and herself out of the eligibility pool at the Hideaway as they sat laughing and talking. Amber nursed a beer as Norris surprisingly drank soda. She patiently waited for him to make his move. He did. Amber confided that she had always wanted to ride in a big truck for a couple of days just to see what it was like. Naturally, Norris told her that he owned one of the biggest and best on the road. Amber acted surprised but accepted his invitation to ride up to the Oakwood fuel stop and check out his big truck and maybe consider riding to New Orleans and back with him.

Amber followed Norris up to the fuel stop where his unit was parked. Amber parked over by the store building and waited for Norris to walk over. Knowing this small town with its day counters and busy bodies, she was not about to pull up on the truck lot and leave her car parked next to Norris's big truck. Folks would say that she lowered herself down to the lot lizard (truck-stop parking-lot working girl) status. Norris read her thoughts and pulled up beside her. He got out, talking a mile a minute. He suddenly stopped talking and cocked his head and listens a minute. "What's my reefer unit doing running?" he asked out loud to himself as well as Amber.

"Just how in the world would I know that, Norris?" she asked.

"Well, that trailer is empty. Unless Lea has been trying to get in touch with me to pick up a load of seafood and sent Milt down to start the reefer unit, I don't know," said Norris, checking his cell phone.

Sure enough, Lea had called him an hour before. He had left his cell phone in his pickup while playing pool at the Hideaway Lounge. "Shit," he said out loud, "I hope she ain't give that load of seafood to Omaha to somebody else," as he frantically dialed Lea's number, knowing he could get a boxed meat backhaul out of Iowa to Beaumont.

Thinking about Anna since he met her, Ryan was wondering if she would call when his cell phone rang. He answered. Anna told him she was alone watching TV, and if he wanted, he could drop by and have a coke or beer.

Ryan always arranged for the girls to come to his place. He never went out hustling his young prey. Anna's beautiful face and body, her dark honey complexion and quick smile captivated his pedophilic mind. She had not resisted his rubbing her leg as she sat by him in the booth. He scribbled the directions to Lynn's place down and said he would be there shortly.

Anna sat on the front doorsteps petting Bo watching the road for Ryan's car. It was getting close to sunset. Mosquitoes and gnats would make staying outside impossible in minutes without industrial-grade insect repellent. She really didn't know for sure what kind of vehicle he drove but was pretty sure it was the ragged out Toyota Corolla parked at Sam's with Kansas license plates.

Ten minutes latter Bo jumped up and looked down the road. Anna could not hear or see the car coming, but Bo knew a strange car was coming down the main road. In a minute, the Toyota Corolla turned into the long driveway to Lynn's house.

Ryan stepped out of the car with a CD in his hand, as promised. Bo decided that Ryan's visit was unwelcome. Standing on the porch between Anna and Ryan, Bo growled a deep throaty teeth-bearing growl warning Ryan to stop and retreat. Anna quickly stepped forward to grab Bo's collar and scold him for being so aggressive. Anna told Ryan to go on inside. Ryan didn't have to be told twice as he stepped around Anna and Bo getting the screen door between him and the dog. Anna followed, leaving Bo on the front porch unhappy with the stranger's incursion into his domain. Anna noticed that he had changed into shorts and muscle shirt. He smelled of expensive shaving lotion. As she thought, "What a great looking guy," he handed her the CD and moved very close to her. He puts his arms around her. She steps in closer thinking he was going kiss her. His hands were fumbling with her halter straps.

Anna, realizing what a terrible mistake she had made by inviting him, knew she must make a phone call as she stepped back and said, "Ryan, wait a minute. I have to go the bathroom. Be back shortly. Get yourself a beer out of the fridge."

Picking up her purse off the bed, she went into the bathroom and locked the door. Turning on the noisy fart fan, Anna removed her cell phone from her purse and punched five and call on the keypad. Thank God for one-touch dialing as Mia answered on the first ring. "Ryan is here, Miss Mia. Please hurry." She hung up before Mia could say another word. She flushed the commode to make Ryan think she had used it in case he was listening. Checking her lipstick in the mirror, she unlocked the door and walked back into the living room and found Ryan sitting at the kitchen bar drinking one of Mr. Lynn's beers. She walked straight to the front door, opened it, and motioned to Bo to come inside. Beside her leg in less than a heartbeat, Bo made up his mind that Ryan was not good company and that he would protect Anna.

"Why did you let that dog in, Anna?" asked Ryan.

"I feel comfortable with him beside me. Don't you like dogs?" asked Anna.

"As a matter of fact I don't particularly care for them, especially that one. He is not friendly."

"Yes he is. I can handle him as good as Mr. Lynn can," said Anna reaching down to pet Bo. The Australian Blue Heeler dog was bred primarily for stock herding. Exceptionally smart and easy to train, the Blue Heeler puts loyalty to its master above its own safety. Bo was exceptionally smart knowing Lynn and Anna as his masters since he was a puppy. Pleasing them was what he lived for. Anna had spent untold hours playing with Bo and training him to do all sorts of chores on the small farm. Bo now stood beside Anna, his eyes watching every move that Ryan made, with his hackles up. Somehow, Bo knew, when Anna opened the door for him to come inside, that Ryan was the reason he was inside. Lynn never allowed him inside the house.

"Why don't you put that dog outside and we can have some fun?" said Ryan getting off barstool.

Bo stepped in front of Anna and lowered his head to the level of his back. Anyone could tell that he was now in the attack mode if provoked or his master told him to do so. Anna replied, "Not until you promise that you will keep your hands off me."

"I thought that's what you wanted," answered Ryan.

"You come out here and start to undress me before you are in the house. What is wrong with you, Ryan? Do you think I'm a whore or what?" Anna asked, now mad at him for being so crude.

"You certainly dress like a girl who likes men and sex. I'm a man and I like women and sex. Here we are together. Now put that dog out and let's have some fun," said Ryan.

"Are you saying I dress like a whore?" asked Anna, now infuriated at the pedophile as she continued, "I'm too old for you, Ryan. You like twelve-year-old girls. I'm seventeen and not a virgin, but I damned sure ain't no whore, big buddy."

"Aw come on, Anna. I didn't drive out here to listen to that crap. Get the dog out and come over here."

"Bo ain't going nowhere. Take your CD and leave, Ryan."

"You throwing me out?"

"Yes. Please leave," said Anna, "I am not going to let you rape me."

"Look, I thought you wanted me to come out here and do a little quickie. I go home, you watch TV, and everybody would be happy," said Ryan.

"If you had come in here acting right you could have spent the whole night with me. But no, you come here trying to undress me before I can close the door, treating me like a whore," said Anna.

"You planned to let me spend the night?" asked Ryan not believing his ears.

"Not now I'm not. You don't know how to treat a girl."

"Let me start over then, Anna."

"No, I'm just not interested anymore. You messed up."

"Let me make this up to you, Anna," said Ryan stepping closer to her.

Bo growled low and deep as he crouched. Ryan looked down at the dog whose hackles were up, eyes turned green with rage, and his quivering lips pulled back to show teeth. Slobber drooled from Bo's mouth as he waited for Anna's command.

"No. Don't come any closer to me, Ryan. If you touch me I'll sic Bo on you."

Lynn was in the checkout line at the convenience store with a suitcase of beer. He was going to get Mia a pack of cigarettes and himself a can of snuff. He noticed Mia talking on the phone in his pickup parked close to door as he stood in line. She abruptly hung up and popped the door open, ran to the door of the store, and busted in, saying, "He's out there. Let's go." Lynn set the beer on an ice cream freezer and ran to the pickup behind Mia. Everyone in the store now wondering what the matter was.

Laying down rubber as Lynn left the store, it was only three or four minutes to his place if he hurried. Mia frantically dialed Lea's number. She too silently thanked the telephone gods for one-touch dialing. Lynn was driving so fast and turning corners she could hardly ride much less use the phone.

After what seemed like twenty minutes and twenty miles Lynn pulled into his driveway. He parked behind the Corolla. Hitting only the middle step on the porch, he was at the door before Mia reached the porch. Hearing Bo inside growling and barking, Lynn knew what was happening before he opened the door.

Ryan heard the pickup as it braked hard to turn into the driveway. "You set me up, you little slut," screamed Ryan, forgetting about Bo as he lunged for Anna. Bo attacked without a command stopping Ryan in his tracks. He stepped back and again moved toward Bo. As he kicked, Bo simply faded to the left and nailed him in the calf of his leg while it was extended. Herding dogs expect to be kicked. Therefore Bo expected Ryan to kick. Pain raced to Ryan's brain before he could get his foot back on the floor. Bo didn't let him get it back on the floor. Ryan tried to stand on one leg and beat the dog off, but tripped and fell backwards. His head hit a rung in the barstool as he fell, adding to his dilemma. Before he could get up, Bo was in his face big-time. Ryan screamed, "Get this dog off me!" as Lynn burst though the door.

Anna was watching. She had made no move to make Bo stop. Ryan's jaw, lower lip, ear, and leg were bleeding all over the carpet. Mia rushed in and pulled Anna away from the fracas, hugging her, asking if she was okay. Lynn made Bo stop and told Ryan to get up and get on the tile floor in the kitchen. Ryan lay there staring at Lynn. When the cowboy boot made contact with Ryan's rib cage, breaking three, he got up as quickly as his wounds would allow him and stood on the tile floor holding on to the kitchen cabinet countertop staring at Lynn seething with rage.

Mia, seeing Ryan was now under control, walked over to the stove behind him. She picked up a cast iron frying pan sitting on the stove. Ryan was watching Lynn. He never knew what hit him as Mia with a two-hand grip on the heavy cast-iron skillet handle hit Ryan as hard as she could above and behind his right ear. The skillet made the gong sound. The stud muffin fell like a one-egg cake, out cold as a wedge.

`Lynn said, "Keep him down till I get some duct tape to tie him up with. Anna, get that dog out of here and start cleaning that blood off the carpet before it dries."

Lynn headed for his pickup to get duct tape out of his toolbox. No experienced trucker with would dare be caught without a roll of duct tape in his big truck and personal vehicle. Lynn was no exception. In the long-haul trucking world, cell phones, whiteout correction fluid, and caller ID rank right on up there with duct tape as absolute necessities.

Milt and Lea arrived as Lynn finished duct taping his hands and ankles together. Lynn did not put any tape over Ryan's mouth like they do in the movies.

Milt rushed over to Ryan lying on the kitchen floor to check him out. Lea went to Mia and asked what happened. Mia told Lea and Milt what was going down when they arrived. Lea turned to Anna noticing she had changed clothes asked, "You thought you would have some fun before you called, and it backfired, didn't it?"

Crying softly and scared to death that Lynn would join in, she hung her head and nodded yes.

"Did he have his way with you, Anna?" Lea asked.

"No ma'am. But he did try to take my clothes off as soon as he got here. I let Bo inside to protect me and went in the bathroom. I called Miss Mia from in the bathroom."

"Looks like Bo did a good job holding him off until we got here," said Lynn.

"We can't stand around here talking. Where is Amber? The Stud Muffin here needs to take a ride," said Mia, her voice now cold and calm. Everyone noticed she sounded like a different person. Lynn looked at Milt and Lea. Lea barely shook her head, but Lynn picked up on it right away.

Lea stepped out on the porch and dialed Amber's cell phone. She answered on the seventh ring. Lea said, "Amber, we have the cargo. Where is Norris?"

"He's in the store getting us some cigarettes." answered Amber. "Did he call you about fifteen minutes ago?"

"Yeah, is he drinking?"

"No. He's being a good boy. I've got him wrapped around my little finger right now. That man has the hots for me."

"Good. Get him away from his truck for about a half an hour at least and we will load our cargo and then you can ride with Norris to New Orleans. Call me when you get him away from the truck. It's almost dark now. We need to roll, Amber," said Lea hanging up.

Lea walked back inside and said, "Amber is getting Norris away from his truck. We can load him up and be ready to put him in Norris's trailer when Amber calls back."

Lynn headed out the front door and backed his pickup up to the front door steps. He went around the house to the barn and got a horse blanket and returned to the house through the kitchen door. It was not completely dark as Lynn and Milt rolled Ryan onto the horse blanket, picked the blanket up with Ryan inside, and loaded him into the pickup backed up to the front porch. Lynn made sure Ryan was covered with the blanket before he slammed the tailgate shut. "We're ready to go when Amber calls," announced Milt as they stood on the front porch.

Mia fired up a cigarette while watching the blanket in Lynn's truck. She was proud of herself that she had cold cocked Ryan with the skillet. Ryan had molested her godchild and ignored her at Sam's that night she and Toby went dancing. Engrossed with her vengeful and unfounded accusations, Mia gloated over the fact that the Stud Muffin was about to get what was coming to him as she took a long drag off of her cigarette.

Lynn checked on Anna. She was still cleaning the carpet. She was still crying, afraid Lynn was going to fire her for messing up. Lynn, upset as he was, asked if she was okay. She tuned up again. Tears started rolling down her cheeks as she answered Lynn, "I only wanted see if he was really like that. He seemed so nice at Sam's, Mr. Lynn. I didn't mean to mess you and Miss Mia up."

"You didn't call like I asked you to do, Anna. You called when you got in trouble. What I want to know is, if he had been nice to you would you have called at all?" asked Lynn.

"Yes sir, I was going to call you."

"When? After you had your fun or what?"

Anna just hung her head. She was expecting to be fired on the spot. She had never seen Mr. Lynn so mad. Miss Mia would probably never let her work for her again either.

Mia had stepped inside and was listening to Lynn's small tirade. She had calmed down now that she had Ryan. Lynn asked Anna, "Are you that hard up to find a boy to date?"

Wiping her eyes with the back of her hand, she looked Lynn straight in the eye answering, "I don't like to date boys, Mr. Lynn. I like men at least five years older than me. Boys are silly and boring."

"You know, Lynn, I got to be the same way when I was about her age and did lots of foolish stuff. Why don't we just let it rest? We got Stud Muffin and no harm is done except to your carpet. Looks like Anna has got that almost got taken care of don't you, baby?" said Mia walking over to Anna and hugging her up and patting her back.

Anna smiling now said softly, "Thanks for understanding, Miss Mia."

Mia slapped her butt and said, "Get this mess cleaned up before we get back."

Lynn hugged Anna before he and Mia went out on the porch. Lea was on the phone talking to Amber. She asked a couple of questions and hung up. "It's time to go." All four of them got into Lynn's pickup. His pickup was a three-door with a small back seat.

It took only twelve minutes to get to the fuel stop and get Ryan inside Norris's trailer and the doors padlocked. As they left the parking lot Lea called Norris and dispatched him to New Orleans for a load to Omaha. She reminded him that the load appointment was for five tomorrow morning. Lea lied to Norris about the appointment time. She just wanted Ryan out of Oakwood as soon as possible.

Mia was adamant about going with Lynn to follow Norris and Amber. Lea and Lynn had discussed this matter briefly. Mia wanted Ryan to stay in the trailer well past Baton Rouge. Ryan would be frozen solid by that time with the freezer unit turned to twenty below zero. Lynn assured Mia that Ryan would be frozen almost to death by the time Norris got down to the big road (I-20) which was only twenty-five minutes away. Lynn wanted to dump Ryan out after about a half-hour in the freezing trailer thinking that would scare him and Toby out of Oakwood. After a lot of talking and arguing, Mia finally agreed to stay behind and be ready to help if they called. Mia and Milt would be on standby while Lea and Lynn made the trip. Milt had a real busy workday tomorrow.

Milt went and got Lea's Suburban while they watched for Norris and Amber. Lynn was afraid that Norris might recognize his pickup following them. Lea's Suburban had a CB and cell phone. Milt got back with the Suburban with a full tank of gas just as Norris and Amber showed up. Norris cranked up the truck and unlocked the passenger door for Amber. He turned on all his lights, bumped all his tires, and checked all his lights as made his way around the rig. He quickly and expertly finished pretriping his rig. He turned the reefer unit off, noticing the temp inside the trailer was eight degrees. Norris put his clothes and stuff in the sleeper, Amber climbed in; Norris laid a clipboard on the steering wheel and started his pretrip report. Next, he fixed his logbook. Norris pushed the red and yellow knobs in on the dash, releasing the air parking brakes on the tractor and trailer and eased the big red International Navistar Eagle off the parking lot.

Norris had not lied to Amber about his rig. His unit was one of the finest rigs International Navistar had ever made. Norris had tastefully added extra chicken lights (the rows of amber lights set in a chrome strip) under the sleeper and doors and several other lights on the back of his trailer to make his unit easily recognizable in the dark to his friends. The floodlights in the parking lot reflected off the polished Alcoa aluminum wheels as Lynn, Mia, and Milt watched Norris ease out of the fuel stop and get the big unit up in the wind.

Behind a farm co-op store they waited a couple of minutes before leaving. Lea stood by Lynn's pick up, kissed her husband goodbye, and whispered into his ear, "Lynn is going to take that man out of there at Lake Charles, maybe before that if Norris will stop." Milt never said a word. He hugged his wife tight and then got in Lynn's pick up and drove away with Mia.

Lynn got under the wheel without asking Lea if he could drive. Lea didn't object; in fact, she expected him to drive. They soon had Norris's trailer lights in view. He would be easy to follow because of the unusual tail light configuration on his trailer.

Amber, sitting in a plush air ride seat, was amazed how nice this truck was on the inside. The only big truck she had ever ridden in was that raggedy-assed old pulpwood truck that her daddy owned. The International Navistar Prosleeper cab was designed for long-haul driver comfort. The Navistar folks didn't miss much in this model. Finally, after looking things over a few minutes, she asked, "Norris, does this thing have a cook stove in here somewhere?'

"Naw it don't, baby, but it's got a microwave and refrigerator right back there behind you in the sleeper compartment," said Norris pleased that she liked his truck. "Get up and take a look around back there."

Amber unfastened her seat belt, lifted the left armrest on her seat, and went into the sleeper compartment. "You can stand up in here. Man, I could really get into traveling like this. This is really nice."

Norris, never taking his eyes off the road, answered, "I live in here more than I live at home. This is my business and I damn sure take good care of my rig. If you don't you won't be in the long-haul business long. When we load this thing with perishable stuff, the shipper and customer expects it there on time and not messed up. You live and prosper by your reputation in this business, Amber. Luck don't cut it out here."

Back in the shotgun seat Amber remarked, "For the life of me I can't get over how smooth this thing rides and how quiet it is in here.

95

I would have thought that you couldn't hear yourself think up in here."

"That's exactly why I bought this particular rig. I drove one at a truck stop demonstration show and I ordered this thing. I spec'd this truck out from the ground up."

"I don't know jack shit about trucks but looks to be like you got it right."

"Thanks. You comfortable over there?"

"Yeah but I'm gonna need to use the bathroom pretty quick though."

"I'm gonna stop and fill my coffee cup in Lake Charles in a few minutes."

"That'll work."

Lynn and Lea were following Norris, making small talk. Lea had been around Lynn since they were teenagers. She never gave it a second thought about getting in the car with him and going on a trip that would last until late in the night or early morning at best. Her husband didn't seem to mind either, even if he did, he didn't say anything. She watched Lynn as he drove and for some reason thought about how good he felt when she hugged him that afternoon behind Amber's shop. She was ashamed for lusting after Lynn, yet jealous of Mia for having him all to herself. She remembered when she dated him in high school. He had kissed her and fondled her some but never tried to go all the way.

"If Norris stops and gets coffee like he usually does in Lake Charles, I will get Ryan out and cut him loose while you watch for me. He usually parks around on the dark side of the convenience store and hangs around and flirts a while with the girls who work in there," said Lynn after the lull in the conversation.

"What if he catches us, Lynn?" asked Lea with apprehension in her voice.

"Everything will be okay, Lea. I'll get Ryan out and put him over there by the trash dumpster and we'll be out of there," said Lynn trying to make her feel better.

"Yeah, but you didn't answer my question, Lynn,"

"I told Amber that every time she got him to stop to keep him inside for at least ten minutes. Amber said if nothing else worked she would make him stop and she would seduce him."

"That's nice of Amber. She can always figure out a way to get some. Don't make her a bad girl as far as I'm concerned," said Lea before she thought, putting her hand to her mouth before continuing, "After all, Norris is a great-looking guy. Mia talked about dating him before she got hooked with you. Bet you didn't know that did you, Lynn."

"Naw, I didn't. I just don't like the man."

"You bedded his ex wife, and he didn't like that. He was trying to get her into rehab and get her back. To put it plain, Lynn, Norris don't like you because you fucked his wife."

"Well, I only did it once. I didn't know they were trying to get back together. She never mentioned it," answered Lynn, glancing at Lea. He had never heard her use the F word.

"Well, Amber may get him straightened out. She is quite pretty when she fixes up."

"I've noticed that myself. If Mia and I were not together I would ask her out."

Feeling a little miffed, Lea brazenly asked, "If Milt and I were not together would you ask me out, Lynn?"

"No. I would not ask you out, Lea. I would take you out and keep you until you said, 'Take me home with you. I would marry you, Lea. You know how I feel about you."

Lea unhooked her seat belt and slid over beside Lynn. She put her arm around him and kissed him on the cheek, his neck, and back on his cheek. She rubbed her boobs against his arm and chest saying, "You know I'd take you up on that offer," and slid back to her side and buckled up.

Chapter 9

Norris hit Interstate 10 and picked his speed up to seventy for a few miles until he came to the exit where he wanted to get off and let Amber pee. He circled around the back of the store building to park on the south side. Three freight haulers each pulling a set of doubles were completely blocking the drive were on that side of the building. Norris had no choice but to pull up behind the freight haulers, go get his coffee, and let Amber do her business. Lynn decided it was just too risky to take Ryan out of the trailer here unless Norris pulled the truck up some more. The rear end of his trailer was in clear view of the fuel islands.

Inside the trailer Ryan's head was killing him. He shivered as he opened his eyes. Inside the reefer trailer was black as midnight under a washtub. Ryan, thinking he was blind, moaned as he tried to rub his eyes with his hands duct-taped together. Not a shred of light filtered inside the reefer trailer as he lay on the floor shaking from the freezing temperature inside the insulated reefer trailer. Ryan found himself in a huge deep freeze, almost soundproof as well as expertly engineered for temperature climate control, a deep-freeze would go to thirty below if necessary. Ryan did not realize that he was in a reefer trailer and thought he was locked in a walk-in beverage cooler. Screaming could not be heard by the trio of freight truck drivers standing beside the trailer shooting the bull before driving off to complete their Baton Rouge-Houston turnaround.

A muscle shirt and pair of shorts is not the proper attire for riding in a reefer trailer with the temp already down below freezing when

Norris killed the small Kubota diesel engine that powered the freezer unit back in Oakwood about an hour ago. Ryan was terrified thinking that if he was in a convenience store he should see a light though the glass doors. Had the lick to his head blinded him? Hurting as bad as it was, it was certainly was a possibility. Ryan screamed again as the three freight haulers rolled out of the parking lot chatting on their CB radios.

He crawled and scooted to the wall on his right and scooted down the wall to the front of the trailer and then down the other side to the rear doors. With taped hands Ryan felt for a door handle or release knob to open the doors. Sorry, no inside door handles. Choking on fear, nearly freezing, his side hurting, the knot on his head killing him, Ryan screamed for help. He moved to the right side off the trailer very close to the doors and sat down. "Why did I go to meet that wetback whore? I've never been that foolish before," cried Ryan as he broke down completely, shaking like a dog shitting peach seeds.

Amber didn't appreciate Norris standing there blatantly flirting with the fat girl working behind the counter. Norris paid for his coffee and Amber's fountain drink and they finally left. Norris climbed up into his truck and immediately said, "I'll be damned. The 'check coolant light' is on."

"Is that bad? asked Amber checking out the flashing light in the dash and hearing the dreaded pinging warning alarm.

"Let me take a look, maybe not," said Norris, already out of the cab and pulling the hood latches. He put his boot in the slot in the polished chrome front bumper, grabbed the indentation on front of the red fiberglass hood, leaned back, and popped the hood. The air clutch on the radiator fan kicked on the thirty-inch diameter six-blade fan as Norris looked for water leaks and tried to remember if he had ever added water or antifreeze to the radiator. He'd had this truck only five months and was certain he hadn't added coolant. He looked at the water reservoir mounted on the firewall. The green liquid was not showing in the glass bulb, indicating the radiator was low on coolant. A small river of water was running from under the truck as Amber pointed out to Norris. "Naw, the air conditioning unit is doing that," he answered.

"Damned shore looks like antifreeze water to me. It's green as grass."

Norris looked down, now realizing this problem was more serious than he thought. Sure enough, the air conditioner was pouring water out as it wrung the humidity out of the Gulf Coast air. As Norris stepped up to the right steering axle tire and looked, sure enough, the green coolant was dripping from the front of the engine. Running under the truck and mixing with the air-conditioning condensation, the coolant turned the water light green as it flowed from under the big truck's right fuel tank.

Norris walked around to the driver's side of the truck, stepped up on the top running board, retrieved a flashlight, and returned to check out the leak. Amber stood back with a cigarette in her lips, arms crossed lussing her breast, as Norris, swearing under his breath, checked out the source of the water leak.

"Shit! The damned water pump has went out on this sucker," said Norris looking at his watch. "I'd bet my ass against a broke plate that you couldn't find somebody that could get a water pump and fix this son-of-a-bitch till in the morning. I might was well call Lea and Milt and let 'em know we're broke down." He walked around to the driver's side and climbed in and dialed Lea's home number. No answer. He dialed her cell phone and watched the coolant temp gauge. Lynn and Lea, across the road in a parking lot watching, already had figured a problem had developed with Norris's truck. Lea answered on the first ring. Listening carefully, she said to try to get somebody out there or call the International dealer in Lake Charles to see if they were still open. A lot of big truck dealership shops are open sixteen and up to twenty-four hours a day. Norris promised to call back no matter how late it was and let them know if they could work on his unit tonight.

Norris got an empty plastic antifreeze jug out of his side box, filled it with water from over at the fuel island, and filled the reservoir with water before he started calling. He explained to Amber that when the water level got lower, the engine would shut down because it has a low-water level shut down built into the system to keep from ruining the engine. He added, "We need a cool place to sit while calling," as he patted her leg. "This truck is still under warranty. If I can find somebody, they will come out and fix this sucker if they can get a water pump. This engine has a great warranty and Detroit Diesel backs it up a hundred per cent. Must've been a bad water pump bearing. Water pumps never fail on a Detroit engine."

Norris was correct. Detroit Diesel Series Sixty engines are legendary for reliability and fuel mileage as well as their low-end torque pulling power under a heavy load. No other diesel truck engine builder on the planet could match the Series 60's performance and reliability. Norris knew this and was aware, as all truckers are, that shit happens. He called the International house and found it open. The night shop foreman instructed Norris to find a place to drop his trailer and bobtail it in, explaining that their drop lot was full. The shop foreman assured him that a mechanic and helper would stay over and get him back on the road.

Norris called Lea back and told her that the International house was going to work on his unit tonight to get him on the road. He was going down to the truck stop and drop his trailer and bobtail to the shop. Norris indicated that if they talked like several hours he and Amber would probably call a cab and get a room and start again in the morning. Lea hesitated before she said, "Okay."

"I need to call and check on Sly, Lynn, and then call Milt and fill him in. Sly is over at Mama's and I ain't called today," said Lea.

Milt rode back to Lynn's house with Mia to get his truck. Mia asked if he would like to get something to eat before he went home. Milt said he had had a big day and better pass, saying that if folks seen just you and me out together the talk would start.

Mia laughed saying, "So what? Let 'em talk. Nothing like changing up partners once in while. You ought to try it sometimes, Milt," as she drove away tickled about making Milt blush.

Faintly hearing a ringing above the radio, Mia touched the button that answered her cell phone and put the sound through the radio speakers. She had the dash-mounted deal allowing her to talk with the phone in the holder. She smiled as she recognized the familiar voice answering, "Hi, Daddy. What going on?" Mia pulled to the shoulder of the road to talk. She and her dad talked for a while before Lea's phone call interrupted Mia's visit with her dad. Promising her dad that she would call him right back, she hung up and opened the line to Lea.

Bo announced Milt's arrival before he recognized him. He patted Bo and played with him for a minute. Milt saw the lights and TV on in Lynn's house as he got in his pickup. Milt decided he ought to check on Anna. He went to the door and knocked. Anna opened the door immediately, wearing nothing but one of Lynn's tee shirts and panties. The tee shirt hung to Anna's knees. He smelled hamburger meat frying on the stove. Anna had a spatula in her hand.

"Is everything all right, Anna? I came to get my pickup and thought I might better check on you," said Milt unable to take his eyes off her beautiful breasts. Her erect nipples pushing the thin cotton tee shirt on out there clearly indicated she wore no bra.

"Yes, everything is all right, Milt," said Anna intentionally leaving the mister off. "Come on in. I'm just fixing me a burger. Can I fix you one?" she asked.

The smell of the fresh ground meat cooking smelled great to Milt who had had nothing to eat since breakfast. She opened the door wider and Milt entered.

"I think I will take you up on your offer, Anna. That meat frying really smells good," said Milt.

"You want one or two burgers, Milt?" asked Anna. Milt noted she had left off the mister this time.

"Two. I'm hungry," said Milt taking a seat at the kitchen bar beside Anna's plate.

"Tea or soda?"

"Tea is fine."

"They get everything taken care of?"

"Ain't heard from them yet. Expecting a call after while."

"Mr. Lynn will take care of everything. Don't worry."

"I'm sure he will," said Milt.

"Maybe after this, Ryan and Toby will leave and never return," said Anna placing Milt's burger patties in the skillet.

"I certainly hope so,"

Anna set a glass of iced tea on the kitchen bar for Milt with a paper towel folded for a napkin. She asked, "Do you want your buns toasted? Mayo or mustard?"

"I'll eat it anyway you fix it," said Milt watching as she reached for the bread in the cabinet. He wondered if the tee shirt was all she was wearing.

Anna looked Milt and asked, "You tired, Milt? Long day, huh?"

"Yeah, a long day."

Anna went to turn off the TV and kicked the CD player on with the same CD that Ryan had brought to her earlier. She walked behind Milt and began to massage his neck and back saying, "This should make you feel better." Anna liked the way he smelled up close, not like some boy wearing half a gallon of shaving lotion and deodorant but like a man. Her rubbing hands spiked his blood pressure up into the 'whoa, wait a minute here' mode. "You like that don't you?" Anna asked softly.

"You better believe I do. You are the only woman that's ever done that besides Lea," admitted Milt.

"That's kinda funny in a way. This afternoon I was a fourteen-year-old girl. Tonight I'm a woman," remarked Anna jokingly as she went to turn the burger patties.

"Yeah, that's right. A very pretty and sexy woman, I might add."

"You think I'm sexy, Milt?"

"Are you joking? You are one of the best-looking women I've ever seen."

Anna was waiting for the patties to finish cooking, wanting to be on the other side of the bar where Milt was. She waited a couple of minutes before taking up the patties and putting them on the buns then setting the plate on the bar in front of Milt. Only Bo noticed the same truck pass in front of the house the third time. When she came to sit at the bar by Milt he jokingly said, "It's my time to rub on you," rubbing her neck and back.

"Eat your burger; then you can rub all you like," Anna said, reaching for his hand and squeezing it just as she removed it. Milt's cell phone rang. His hand was now rubbing on Anna's naked thigh. The phone rang again. Bo turned his head toward Milt's pickup. Milt had laid the phone on the seat of his pickup before he went to check on Anna. Bo raised his head and listened. That truck was passing again.

Milt gobbled his burgers down and waited for Anna to finish. "You in a hurry?" she asked.

"No, I was hungry."

"I'm finished now," Anna said, wiping her mouth and sliding off the barstool. Milt pulled her to him. She grinned as she unsnapped the buttons on his cowboy shirt and run her hand through the hair on his chest.

Kissing her neck, he whispered, "On the couch or in the bedroom," while running his hands up her ribs until he reached her breast. As he caressed both of them Anna stepped closer, put her hand behind Milt's neck, pulled his head down, and kisses him full on the mouth. She held him tight as she explored his tonsils with her probing tongue. Finally she broke away and whispered, "In the bedroom," leading him to the room she slept in when she slept over.

Anna never bothered to turn the light on. She helped her partner undress and let him take off her tee shirt.

Bo watched the truck pull into the driveway and stop down at the road. Out of curiosity he watched but did not bark or move off the porch. In Anna's room Milt was putting on his clothes when Lynn's phone rang. Anna slipped her tee shirt on and answered it. Mia didn't ask if Milt was there; she simply asked to speak to Milt.

Milt took the phone and said, "Hello."

"You finishing what Ryan started earlier or what?" asked Mia.

"What do you mean? I checked on her, and she offered me a burger. I stayed to eat. I was walking out the door when the phone rang. Why you calling for me anyhow?"

"Lea has been trying to call you for an half an hour. She called me and I told her I would find you if I could. Well, your truck was still out here, and I found you. We got problems in Lake Charles."

"What the matter?"

"Dickhead's truck blew a water pump. He's got it in the shop but it'll be about five hours before its ready. Before you call Lea, I need to talk you. I'm sitting at the end of Lynn's driveway."

"Come on up. I'm leaving anyhow," said Milt, wondering what her problem was as he hung up.

Milt said bye to Anna, slapping her on her butt and rubbing the back of his hand across her breast as he walked out. Mia was parked beside his truck waiting. He got in Mia's Yukon asking, "What's wrong?"

"Nothing really. Your wife leaves with my boyfriend, and you are over here fooling around with Anna. I can live with that, but I need a favor."

"Name it," said Milt, sensing that Mia knew he had just bedded Anna. Was she going to blackmail him or what?

Running her tongue over her lips before she asked, "I need you to go with me to Lake Charles."

"Lynn and Lea are down there. Can't they handle that?"

"No. I want to be sure Ryan doesn't come back to Oakwood. Lea said that according to Amber, Norris has not turned that freezer back on. Lea called him and told him to get that trailer to thirty below zero because they wouldn't load him if the temp wasn't down to specs. And Norris ain't turned that freezer on yet."

"What you want me to do?"

"You and me are going to Lake Charles, and you are going to turn that freezer unit back on down to maximum low temp while his truck is in the shop," said Mia. She casually rubbed his thigh higher up than she should, as she continued, "Next time, try to keep it in the family or in your britches, Big Boy. I didn't know you were shopping around. But don't worry, I won't tell Lea," said Mia, nailing his ass to the cross as she backed up, turned, and drove down the lane to the highway, not giving Milt a choice.

"Don't tell me this shit, bro. I gotta be in New Orleans by five in the morning," said Norris to the shop foreman. "They's gotta be a water pump that'll fit that engine closer than Houston. I'll be here all damn day tomorrow twiddling my thumbs, waiting for that thang to get here. Then ya'll gonna drag ass around all evening putting it on there."

"Well, Norris that's about the best we can do. We order it now. Be here about dinnertime tomorrow. Oughta have you out before six," said the gray-headed man seeming totally unconcerned if the truck engine ever got fixed. He heard a similar rendition of a trucker's 'got to be somewhere story' every evening he had worked here for the last twelve years. "We're fixing to close till seven. Go on up to the truck stop and be back in the morning. I'll order the water pump right now, Norris," said the shop foreman as he turned to work on some paper work.

Norris stormed out of the truck shop. Norris slammed the door pretty hard when he got in his truck. Amber didn't have to ask what was wrong. It was well past midnight; Norris was in a bad mood until Amber replied, "What's wrong with you? This will just give us more time to party. Let's go get a drink somewhere and worry about this thing tomorrow."

Norris turned to Amber and said, "There's a motel and bar not far from here. Let's go."

"What about going back to the truck stop and turning that freezer unit on like Lea asked?" said Amber.

"That trailer will be plenty cold when I get to the Dome (New Orleans) tomorrow night if I turn it on before I leave."

Mia, running almost eighty down the two-lane road towards Lake Charles, had Milt a might edgy. Lea told her the trailer was dollied down at the truck stop, and Amber and Norris were partying down. Lea indicated that Amber and Norris had rented a motel and the truck wouldn't be fixed until late afternoon tomorrow.

"Call Lea and tell her that me and her is going to swap places when we get there. I want to see this through. I'll arrange to be off tomorrow. First, you and me are going to turn that freezer unit back on. Tell Lea we will meet them at the motel where Norris and Amber are staying. Lynn and I will take care of the rest of this ourselves," said Mia, closing the subject for debate as she handed Milt the telephone.

Milt relayed the message and told them that they were already on the way. They agreed to meet.

Lea related what the new plan was to Lynn as they sit in Lea's Suburban on the opposite side of the motel parking lot watching the bar and listening to the radio. She phoned Amber and filled her in on the latest move.

"You know, Lynn, I was sort of looking forward to staying out all night with you and tomorrow. In a way, this has been nice to talk to you and all."

"Yeah, Lea, I know. You stay and we probably will get around to doing things that we'd regret later. If Milt knew we had been messing around he would kill me," said Lynn watching her reaction closely.

He knew she was willing right now, and he wanted to hold her and make love to here more than he ever had another woman.

"You know something?"

"What?"

"I've never had sex with anybody but Milt, Lynn."

"Dog gone, you are still a semi-virgin ain't you?"

"I've acted shameless with you tonight."

"Naw, that don't make you a bad girl, just sexy," said Lynn as he scooted over in the seat and hugged her. Lea hugged back and nibbled on his ear. She could feel his hand now on her bare back, rubbing, feeling, and searching. Lynn was kissing her neck and biting her ear. His hand was now down inside the waistband of her shorts caressing her firm buttocks.

"Are you going to before they get here or wait another fifteen years?" said Lea undoing the buckle on his jeans. The windows were almost fogged over as Lynn pulled Lea's shorts down. She helped him shuck his jeans and pulled his shorts down. As she kicked her shorts off her ankles Lea lay back and pulled Lynn down on top of her. She realized why Mia had let him move in as she took his manhood in her hand to guide him.

Twenty minutes later, Lea asked, "Is this going to mess up you and Mia's relationship, Lynn?"

"Not unless you tell her. Why?"

"I just wondered. I damn shore ain't going to tell her. I plan to get some more of this real soon. Will you give it to me?" asked Lea rubbing his crotch and giggling like a teenage girl.

"Yeah, if you can arrange not to get caught. You can always drive out of town a good ways and meet me when I'm in my big truck," said Lynn.

"I always know where Milt is working. No problem. Let him have his jollies. I'm going to have mine. If I find out that he has been doing his running around on me all along, I may put that ass in the road. Would have done it already but he is good in bed," said Lea still giggling.

"They ought to be here pretty quick."

"I sure wish they wasn't coming so we could maybe get us a room and finish what we started. Don't you?" asked Lea checking her makeup and adjusting her clothes.

"Yeah, next time we'll just have to start earlier, "answered Lynn as Lea's cell phone started ringing.

Amber and Norris found a good pool game going in the small bar across from the motel. Eight ball, at ten a game. They both watched the players, carefully analyzing their weakness and strengths. It was their joint decision to sit and drink a few beers and watch.

The winning player so far was a young guy on the long side of twenty-three, crew cut brown hair, hazel eyes, tall slender Marine drill-sergeant body, and a great smile with flawless teeth. He was wearing a red faded muscle shirt, golfing shorts, and pair of heavy tire-tread sandals with huge brass buckles. It became apparent when his buddy told his competition that they built and maintained radio and cell phone towers why this young man was in perfect physical condition.

Amber watched him hand two shooters in a row their ass on a plate. In both instances, he allowed them one shot with a horrible leave. Amber got up and put her money on the rail indicating she was challenging the winner in the second game.

"This is for ten a game. You sure you want to play?" asked the young man politely.

"She can't wait," answered Norris for her as he sipped his longneck.

The young man didn't drop a ball on the break. A lard-ass used car salesman type guy came very close to beating the young tower builder. The next game he made quick work of an offshore oilfield worker.

Surprisingly the bar sported a great selection of pool cues and the table was in excellent shape. The bar owner was a big pool shooter himself but not here tonight. Amber selected her cue and chalked it carefully while everyone watched the game. When the eight ball dropped, she stood back until the money changed hands, then tight racked the balls and stood back waiting for the tower builder to break. He pumped his cue stick five times before he struck the cue ball with the velocity of a bullet. The white ball went airborne and jumped the table.

Someone retrieved the ball and handed it to the tower builder. Amber walked over and reached for the ball. He pulled it back. "You lose break and game. Gimmie the ball and ten dollars, Sport," said Amber.

"Bullshit," said the tower builder, walking to the end of the table, racking the balls, and getting ready to break again. Amber watched dumbfounded.

On his third pump, the Cajun bartender picked the cue ball up and said, "Off the table. You lose. This is not where high school kids play, son. Pay the lady now or get out." The Cajun people do have a way of explaining everything so even a small child can understand it perfectly the first time.

The tall tower builder handed Amber a ten spot and the cue ball saying curtly, "Don't dare miss a shot, little lady." Amber looked at him a full minute, then smiled. She could drive a cue ball harder than most men. Amber was still hard as a rock and in excellent condition. This was the game she liked to play. Every eye in the house saw that the tower builder was in serious trouble when the cue ball waded into the tight-racked numbered balls with the velocity of a Stinger missile. Three balls fell, two solid colors and one stripe. Glancing around the table at the small-number balls, she began a series of shots that would have been worthy of a TV show.

Three games later Amber sensed a tension growing because she was beating some good local pool players. They were already mouthing off to Norris as they watched her. She never missed a single shot in three games. Amber quietly told Norris it was time to cut out before trouble started. Amber forfeited and left with Norris to their room to do some real partying.

Amber hugged Norris as they walked to their room. She was beginning to really like him. He had not mentioned his lush ex-wife not the first time. Amber liked his manners and thought to herself, "Shit, this is a great-looking man. If he can make good whoopee I may get serious about him. Sam just ain't cutting it lately." She rubbed Norris's butt as they made their way to their room. She was praying that Norris didn't decide to go down to check on his trailer. Unknown to Amber was the fact that Norris did not drink and drive his big truck. Period. After the longnecks, Norris would take at least an eight-hour break. He wouldn't dare move the big rig sitting outside the motel door until up in the middle of the morning. In Louisiana, as well as in most states, a DWI/DUI in a big truck will get the perpetrator hard time and he'd probably never be eligible to hold another class A CDL, forever ending his driving career.

Amber's worrying never showed. She felt good about her budding relationship with Norris, and she had actually enjoyed riding with him so for. Before she left home and went out on her own, she was already aware that trucks do break down. This experience was no great surprise to her, remembering how her daddy's old raggedy-assed pulpwood truck swallowed its tongue at least once a week. She was worried that Ryan would not make it out of the reefer trailer before Mia and Milt got here. She had to call now and tell Lynn to get that man out of that trailer.

While Norris was taking a shower and shaving, Amber stepped outside and called Lea. "Y'all got the man out of that trailer yet?" asked Amber.

"Not yet," answered Lea in a bubbly voice laced with unconcern and giddiness. Amber instantly knew what was going on with Lea and Lynn. She had watched Lea out the window yesterday afternoon, knowing something was brewing that was not kosher.

"Get your asses out yonder to that truck stop and get Ryan out of that trailer before we all wind up in the stout house. This shit has gone far enough as far as I'm concerned. I ain't gonna to do no time for this," said Amber emphatically stung by the way Lea had trivialized what they were here to do. "Mia is going to get us all in trouble with her vengeance, Lea. You and Lynn get on over there and get the stud muffin out of there and turn his sorry ass loose," continued Amber.

Biting her lip and realizing finally what drastic steps they had actually taken outside the law Lea softly said, "You are right, Amber. We are on our way now. I'll call you when we get it done," hanging up without out a goodbye.

Realizing that while she and Lynn were making out like teenagers and not taking care of business like they all had agreed on, Lea panicked. Realizing that the trailer had been at the truck stop over an hour while she and Lynn were making out she literally screamed at Lynn, "Get to that trailer before Milt and Mia get here. We got to turn that man loose before Mia gets here, Lynn. Mia intends to freeze that man to death in our trailer and dump him on the way to New Orleans."

The Suburban engine was already running with the air conditioner turned to max. Lynn dropped the selector into to drive and made a run to the truck stop. No one paid any attention to them as they cruised the lot, looking for Norris trailer. Parked on the drop line pad on the back row Lynn pulled up to the nose of the reefer. Lynn walked to the back of the trailer to unlock the doors. To his surprise, the padlock was unlocked. He quickly opened the door and shined his small flashlight inside the trailer. He pulls himself up into the trailer to get a better look. To his amazement, Ryan was not inside. "How can this be?" he asked aloud to himself.

Lynn jumped to the ground looking around and carefully shutting the doors. He walked along the board fence at the back of the parking lot not ten feet from the back of the trailer. The grass was freshly mown and all the litter picked up. Standing there under the floodlights of the parking lot lights with every big truck at high idle running its air conditioners, Lynn could not imagine what had happened to Ryan. Four people knew that Ryan was in this trailer when it left Oakwood— well five, including Anna. Amber had been with Norris all this time and he hadn't opened the doors to found him. Amber would have called if Norris had found Ryan in his trailer

He went back to the Suburban and drove away from the trailer, looking carefully to see if anyone was watching him leave. Lynn pulled to the four-wheeler parking lot in front of the truck stop, put the Suburban in park letting the engine run with the air conditioner still on max. Lea asked, "You get him out of there?"

"I damned sure didn't. He ain't in there and the door was unlocked."

"What does that mean, Lynn?"

"What it means is that when he come to, he made enough racket that somebody heard him and got him out of there."

"So what?"

"If that's the case, every lawman in southwest Louisiana is looking for all of us right now. That's what it means."

"All we wanted to do was scare him and make him leave," answered Lea, now crying softly. We should have let my Daddy take care of this through the law."

"I ain't got a clue about where he is now."

"I'm calling Amber."

"No. Just sit quiet a minute and let me think about this. Okay?"

"Okay," said Lea sliding up to Lynn, expecting him to comfort her.

"Lea, your husband is due here any minute with Mia. They could be watching us. Mia is a very clever person, Lea," said Lynn, softly patting her thigh and looking to see if her could spot Mia's Yukon.

"My God, I don't know what's wrong with me, Lynn. I just want this behind us tonight without harming that man and to go home," wailed Lea.

"Everything is gonna be fine, Lea. Just let me sort this thing out for a few minutes," said Lynn squinting his eyes as he looked straight ahead, not seeing anything.

In a moment, Lynn turned and looked at her like she was a stranger. His eye lines and skewed mouth announced danger and anger. He looked at Lea, never breaking eye contact, for a full minute.

"What is it, Lynn?" asked Lea, now very uncomfortable thinking in the back of her mind, "Here is why he has never married. The real Lynn is about to manifest himself to me and here I am with him by myself."

"Listen to me for a minute, Lea," reasoned Lynn. "Amber and Norris have been together since they left Oakwood."

"Yes."

"We watched them leave with Ryan in the trailer. Right?"

"You know that's right, Lynn. Why are you asking me these questions that we both already know the answers?"

"Me and you have been together and in contact with everybody by cell phone. Right?"

"Mia and Milt were in Oakwood but are due here any minute if they ain't already here somewhere."

"That's right, Lynn. What are you trying to say?"

"Milt agreed to let the man go and just scare the shit out him. That right?"

"You heard him as well as I did, Lynn. What is your point?"

"My point is that Mia knows where that man is, damn it to hell. She's is the only person left who could possibly know. She's cunning and clever."

"How on earth could she get that done?"

113

"Here is the long and short of this whole deal: if Ryan made enough noise in that trailer to be heard and someone let him out, that's one possibility but the padlock is not broke, just unlocked. If Ryan didn't get someone to open that door, then Mia did."

Lea, now sitting up straight, wiped the tears from her eyes as she finally comprehended what her recent lover laid on her. Shaking her head she asked, "What do you think, Lynn? All this is still a little iffy, ain't it?"

"We're still okay as long as the law don't get involved. They would be watching the trailer if they were and already be all over us by now, so we can assume the law don't know nothing about it yet."

"Well, that just leaves Mia, don't it?" said Lea.

"I'm afraid that's about the way it stands, pretty woman," said Lynn feeling good about his logic.

"You don't reckon that Mia some way got Milt to help her?" asked Lea.

"Naw, Milt wouldn't do that after he agreed to let the man go."

"Mia can be very persuasive and will stoop to anything to get what she wants, Lynn. You know that as well as I do."

"Meaning what?"

"She could be messing around with my husband and blackmailing him or something."

"Bullshit. Get that out of your mind. Milt is the last man on earth she would hit on. She knows that you would be on to that before it got started. Besides that, he was in Oakwood and now on his way down here."

"What we gonna do then?"

"When she gets here, I will confront her. It has to be her if somebody didn't hear the man and let him out."

"How can we find out for sure?"

"Just play it by ear for a while and see how she reacts when she finds out the reefer unit ain't running. Let's watch for them. Let me park so we can watch for them and keep an eye on that trailer, okay."

"Sounds good to me, Lynn. You want a cup of coffee? I'm going inside to use the rest room," said Lea opening the door and getting her purse.

"Yeah. Black is fine."

Chapter 10

Waiting never set well with Lynn. He and Lea had taken only a couple of sips of the hot coffee when Mia's Yukon rolled into the parking lot. Mia headed to the drop line to check out Norris's trailer. She nosed the Yukon up to the front of the trailer and got out with Milt. Lynn and Lea watched as Milt and Mia had a conversation before he started the reefer unit. As Milt was checking the oil and fuel level in the reefer unit's tank, Mia walked to the back of the trailer. Seeing the padlock unlocked she smiled briefly and pushed the padlock until it clicked locking the empty trailer.

Walking back to the front of the trailer, she heard Milt start the reefer unit. He was adjusting the temp as she walked up behind him. Jealousy consumed Lea as she watched Mia stand on her tiptoes and hug her husband cheek to cheek, then get in the Yukon.

Lea looked at Lynn as he glanced briefly at her and shrugged his shoulders. "Let's go see our mates, Lynn, and see what's going on," said Lea.

"Yeah, let's go. Don't let on that we are suspicious of them in any way," said Lynn. "I need to check on something and then I'll know for sure what's going on. I think I already know the answer, though."

"Whatcha talking about?"

"If I find what I am sure I'll find I'm afraid your friend is messing up," said Lynn, looking at Lea and knowing her world was tilting right before her eyes.

"Well, let's go. I'm about ready for a change anyhow," said Lea rubbing his thigh. "I'm ready to get this whole mess over with tonight."

Lynn slipped the Suburban in reverse, backed out, and returned to the drop pad. Mia and Milt were in deep conversation when they noticed Lynn drive up.

Everyone got out and Mia commented, "Well, I got Lynn to turn that freezer down as low as it would go. That bastard in there will be frozen stiff in two hours. Then we will follow Norris and Amber and dump his ass somewhere."

Lynn looked at Mia, thinking, "This pretty woman has lost it. Not a shred of remorse about killing somebody and dumping his body like it was yesterday's garbage."

"Mia, are you sure you want to go freeze this man to death and dump him?" asked Lynn.

"Dammed right I do. He molested Sly and four more young girls. That child- molesting bastard oughta be hung," snarled Mia.

Lynn shook his head and started to the back of the reefer with Lea following him.

"Where are you going?" asked Mia.

"I'm going to check to make sure the trailer is locked," replied Lynn walking down the side of the trailer.

"Yeah, that's a good idea. Don't need somebody to open it looking for something to steal," said Mia.

The parking lot lights were swarmed with a million bugs. The humid air on the hot summer night was stifling as Lynn looked at the locked padlock on the trailer. He knew that she had set all of them up to get at Ryan. Lea had told Lynn that Ryan had snubbed her at Sam's the night that she and Toby went dancing. Lynn looked at Lea, then Milt, and finally at Mia for a long minute. He walked toward the front of the trailer and killed the reefer unit engine.

"What the hell you think you are doing?" screamed Mia.

"Trying to keep all of us out of the penitentiary," said Lynn, walking back to the rear of the trailer digging his keys out of his jeans followed by everyone else.

"I want you to see this man one more time, Mia, before you kill him."

"I don't want to see him and don't unlock that door," screamed Mia.

Lynn, ignoring her, already had his key in the lock and unlocked the padlock. He opened the doors of the trailer. Cold air rushing out of the trailer meeting the hot humid air formed fog so thick Lynn could barely see Mia or Lea.

Mia grabbed the left door and tried to slam it shut. Lynn stopped the slam easily with his left hand and shinned his flashlight and it into the empty trailer with his right hand.

"Why don't you tell us where Ryan is, Mia?" demanded Lynn, not really looking inside the trailer, knowing full well it was empty. Milt stepped closer and took the flashlight searched the inside for Ryan.

"Where is Ryan?" asked Milt, looking at Mia, then his wife.

"That's a good question, Mia. Where is Ryan? You had somebody get him out of there. Where is he?" asked Lynn now all up in her face.

"You think I know where he is?" she answered.

"I know damned well you know. Tell me so I can get him and turn him loose before we all get into serious trouble, woman!" screamed Lynn right into her face nose to nose.

"Why don't you carry your wimpy ass back to Oakwood, buddy? Milt and I will take care of this. Let's go, Milt," said Mia as she headed to her truck. Milt simply shrugged and followed her like a puppy, leaving Lynn and Lea standing there wondering what in world had come over Milt.

Stung to the core, Lea looked at Lynn for help. He shook his head, shrugged, and indicated they go to the Suburban. When they got in Lea asked, "What in the world is wrong with Milt, Lynn?"

"Sorry, pretty woman, but it ain't looking too good for either one of us," answered Lynn. "We may as well head on toward the house. You ready?"

"Yeah, I guess so. Man, has this turned out to be a helluva weird day or what?" remarked Lea.

"I would never have thought that she would take it this far. How about you? You know Mia better than anyone," said Lynn.

"I don't even know my husband or her, Lynn," said Lea, tuning up to cry.

Lynn slid over and hugged Lea. She responded by hugging him back and softy crying as he held her close. Lynn was fit to be tied. He realized his conniving lady friend had used him and Milt. Everything could be easily traced back to them if Mia followed through on her plan. Lynn dialed Amber, realizing it was after two in the morning. He let the phone ring and ring. No answer. Amber's phone ringer was turned off. She was partying down with Norris. After numerous tries, Lynn finally conceded defeat and headed toward Oakwood without Lea's consent.

Obeying her bladder's urgent request for immediate relief, Amber checked her missed calls sitting on the commode in the motel bathroom. Seeing that Lynn had been trying numerous times to reach her, she hurriedly slipped on her jeans and shirt and grabbed her purse. Norris lay on the bed naked as the day he was born, sleeping as if he was drugged. Taking no chance of waking him, she put the motel room key in her purse before stepping outside. She eased the door shut and frantically dialed Lynn's cell phone. Digging in her purse for her cigarettes and lighter, Lea answered before the first ring was completed.

Lea quickly brought Amber up to speed about Ryan missing out of the trailer. Lynn pulled onto the exit ramp and stopped, indicating that he wanted to talk to Amber when she finished. Amber asked, "Where's Mia and Milt?"

"We don't have a clue," was Lea's answer.

"You're bullshitting me, Lea. You mean to tell me that you and Lynn just let 'em just drive off and leave us holding the bag?" hissed Amber.

"What could we do? Mia had her own plan from the start, so it seems," answered Lea, "Here is Lynn. Let him tell you about it." Lea handed Lynn the phone, slid up closer to him, and put her ear next to Lynn's, trying to hear Amber as she talked. Lynn realizing what she was doing cocked the phone so she also could hear Amber's tirade. With everything that happened tonight, she wasn't feeling guilty about herself and Lynn.

"Yeah I know we got to find Ryan, Amber. Looks like she's dead set on freezing that man to death. Do you know of anyone with a reefer trailer that she knows besides me and Norris?" asked Lynn already knowing her answer.

"I sure don't. Do you? What about Lea. She oughta know."

"She don't know anyone as far as I know, Amber," Lea said into the phone as Lynn held it for her.

Amber finally getting her cigarette lit, responded, "We need to find that man. She knows where he is if she ain't done had him killed already.

"We are going to look for them around here the rest of the night and into the morning. Stay with Norris and try to eavesdrop on all his calls if you can. Mia might have enlisted Norris to help her in some way and us not know about it. We will be in touch. Call us about six if you are up, okay?" asked Lynn.

"Don't fog up them windows in that Suburban no more like that, Lynn. Get you a motel room. Y'all ain't no teenagers," said Amber laughing as she rung off.

"So Amber knows," said Lea.

"She won't say nothing," answered Lynn.

"I really don't give a damn right now," said Lea as she snuggled up to him and bit his ear playfully, then slid back to her side of seat. Lynn pulled up to the stop sign, hooked a left, and headed back east across the Calcasieu River to Lake Charles, looking for the needle in the haystack.

Mia pulled out of the parking lot with Milt heading east toward Lafayette. The early in the morning traffic was light on I-10. Lots of tankers and line haul freight trucks that made nightly scheduled runs, hardly any four-wheeler traffic. Mia was seething with anger, wondering how Lynn had figured out her double-cross so quickly. Lea and Amber knew everything by now. Milt watched her as she lit a cigarette. He knew he had to get away from this woman before she got him into even more trouble.

"Pull in to the next place that's open, Mia," said Milt. "I need to use the restroom and get a cup of coffee. Where are we going anyway?"

"Lafayette, right now. Then we are going to get a motel and wait a while. We are going to have a pretty good wait."

"Bullshit. I need to get to the house. Tomorrow is payday. Me and Lea have to be there to settle up with everyone. Turn this thing around and take me to my pickup."

"You don't want to spend the day with me?" asked Mia, now full of herself for making him walk away from Lea and leave with her back at the truck stop.

"No, I don't. Turn around and take me to my truck."

"I want you to help me, Milt. I wouldn't want you and Lea to have problems because of Anna."

"I'll worry about that when time comes. I got a company to run and people to pay today. You'll just have to get whoever took Ryan out of Norris's trailer for you to help you with your plan."

"Okay, I'll take you home but this afternoon I want you to meet me in Lafayette and we will put all this behind us tonight."

"That might work. But get me to the house right now."

Mia wet her lips, realizing she had not completely lost him yet as she reached over, rubbed his thigh, and cooed, "Sure, Milt. Whatever you want."

Milt unfolded his phone and dialed his wife. Lea answered on the third ring noticing that her husband sounded tired and beat. Milt opened with, "Lea, I'm on my way to the house. Where are y'all at, Baby?"

Lea answered, "Still in Lake Charles. Why?"

"Find a place and wait up on me. I want to ride home with you," said Milt.

Lea could tell from the tone of her husband's voice that something was terribly wrong. She had lived half her life with him and could read him like a book. As she listened her hands began to shake and lips began to tremble. Tears were welling in her eyes as he suggested a meeting place.

"We ain't too far away. Be there in a short-short. Bye," said Milt and turning to Mia and giving her direction to their rendezvous.

"When we get there, you get out. I'm leaving. I'm not in the mood to get into a knock-down and drag-out with Lea and Lynn. What gets me is that you above all should want that bastard punished for what he did to Sly, Milt. I just don't understand you or Lea."

"You damned near killed the man with that skillet. We done froze his ass off already. Now you want to kill him. What in the name of God is the matter with you, woman? Has anyone told you lately that it is against the law to kill folks? Whether you think they need killing or not, it is still against the law. What business is it of yours when you get right down to it, anyhow? Sly belongs to me and Lea. True, you are Sly's godmother but you are way out of line on this one, Mia. Besides all else, Sly said he didn't bother her and brushed off his advances. I believe my daughter. She's never lied to us before. Now you tell me where Ryan is so we can go get him and turn him loose."

"Like hell I will. I'm finishing what I started," snarled Mia, "I'm not telling you where he is, so can it. That pedophiling son of bitch has molested his last little girl. The law won't do nothing about it, but I damn sure will."

Sitting beside Mia, Milt's temper flared to the point of hauling off and jack slapping the shit of her. He had never hit a woman. His twenty-four carat Cajun redneck upbringing strictly forbade even thinking about hitting a woman in anger. Very close to the meltdown point, Milt's patience had worn thin as frog hair with Mia. He glanced at her finally realizing she had used all of them to get Ryan out of Oakwood. She intended to follow through with her plan even as doubts were expressed day before yesterday.

"Why am I helping set up Norris? He is one of my best owner-operators, as good as Lynn, or anyone one else. How did I let this bitch talk all of us into this mess is beyond me. Why is my wife riding around with Lynn all night? What in the hell is wrong with me for even allowing all this shit to get started? A real good yard dog ass-whipping would have worked fine on ole Ryan," thought Milt. He told Mia, "Mash on it, I'm ready to get to the house."

At the same fuel stop that Norris and Amber found the water pump going out, Mia pulled into the parking lot. Lynn was standing behind the Suburban waiting on her expecting her to let him ride with her. Maybe he could find out something from her. As soon as Milt shut the door, Mia burned rubber leaving making sure she lost all of them. Milt stood watching her leave, now wishing he had whipped her ass. He and Lynn turned and walked over to Lea's Suburban and got in. Milt indicated that he wanted Lynn to drive. Lea knew Milt was fighting mad, hoping he wouldn't start in on Lynn and herself.

"That bitch won't tell me where Ryan is or who helped her get him out of the trailer. If she ever shows up at the house again I swear I'll whip her no good-ass. You hear me, Lea?" said Milt looking at Lynn, expecting him to say something in Mia's defense.

121

Lynn looked at Milt and nodded in agreement, then put the Suburban in the road to Oakwood.

"Yeah, Milt. I hear you. I don't want Sly around her anymore, period," answered Lea near hysteria. She waited for her husband to start in on her, dreading a tongue-lashing in front of Lynn. Her husband was right to be mad about everything. She had not a leg to stand on if he started in on both of them. Ten minutes ago she wouldn't have cared. Right now she saw her husband mad and hurt. Lea realized that Milt loved her and Sly more than anything. Her infidelity gnawed at the gold band on her left hand as the fingers of her right hand spun the gold band on her third left hand finger unconsciously. Mortified about her indiscretion and knowing that if Amber knew about Lynn and herself, the possibility that Milt finding out loomed very real, really soon.

Teary eyed, Lea stared straight ahead into the predawn darkness thinking about how her own safe and secure world had been turned upside down since the day that Mia come by her house to borrow that cowboy hat to go on a date with Lynn. Close as sisters, Lea and Mia had never had a problem they could not sit down, talk about it, and solve it. Mia for some odd reason had lost all rationality. What was her obsession? What had Ryan actually done to her? Her instinct told her to ask Milt and Lynn to call and get the authorities involved before something really bad happened. Milt's present temperament overrode even opening her mouth. Lynn pushed the suburban hard for Oakwood as himself and his passengers stared into to the dawning light.

Mia, nervous as a harlot in church, grabbed her cell phone as soon as she was certain no one was following her and made a call. The man on the other end was not overjoyed talking to one of the prettiest women on the Gulf Coast before dawn. In fact he was gruff and short with Mia. She bored in, asking all the questions and getting assurance that everything was under control and on schedule. She asked again when and where she was to meet him. He told her to meet him at the truck stop in Henderson at nine o'clock PM. Assured that everything was under control Mia headed to Lafayette listening to the radio and chain smoking. "I'll teach that bastard to turn me off when I'm making my play. No man will put me down like he did at Sam's. I can't wait to throw his low-bred frozen ass to the gators," screamed Mia into the windshield of the Yukon. The windshield never replied, it just kept stopping bugs. The news on the radio was telling about another suicide bomber in Israel.

Amber never went back to bed after talking to Lea and Milt. Drugs got her busted a couple of times on the left coast. Being in the stout house even for a night cropped a bad memory. Amber had really begun to like Norris. He was a lot of fun to be with and liked to party. Her concern was what Mia was up to now that she had Ryan out of Norris's trailer. Amber stood leaning over the railing in front of her room as she lit another cigarette. "I'll whip that bitch's ass when I see her, damn it to hell. I ain't getting in no trouble on the account of her sorry ass," said Amber aloud as she dialed Lea's cell phone.

Lea answered on the first ring. Amber told her exactly what she felt about the deal. Wholeheartedly agreeing with Amber, Lea assured her that they would find where Ryan was and release him if possible. No one had a clue who helped Mia carry out her beguiled plan.

Chapter 11

He worked quickly and expertly, wearing a pair of loose-fitting coveralls, a baseball cap with a Caterpillar logo and wore a new pair of black rubber chemical resistant gloves like a tanker truck driver uses. The big guy roughly removed Ryan's muscle shirt, his shorts, his tennis shoes and socks, his watch, and his high school class ring, carefully putting all the items into a plastic garbage bag. Duct tape was removed from Ryan's ankles and wrist last, taking hair with it. With every scrap of duct tape placed in the garbage bag, the big guy carefully examined Ryan again, finding nothing else remaining to remove.

Ryan was so cold and depressed he could put up no physical resistance but to mumble, "I didn't bother her," repeatedly. He begged the man to release him. His sobbing pleas fell on deaf ears as the man took the plastic bag and jumped out of the trailer slamming and locking the doors.

Ryan crawled to the doors clawing on the plywood attached to the inside of the doors. His fingers were already a bloody pulp from clawing on the doors. His screams and hysteria were masked inside the insulated trailer. "Who was that man? Why did they take me out of one trailer and put me into another one? Why is she having this done to me?" he cried as he crawled to the right side of the trailer and sat down. Convulsions all but paralyzed his body. With great effort, he pulled his legs up and hugged his legs tightly with his arms trying to fight off the cold. Ryan heard the motor start again and the polar air was now blowing extraordinarily cold. He felt the trailer moving. He told himself, "Toby will find me."

Slowly easing off the parking lot, the big red tractor and trailer pulled into the street and a block away swung onto the eastbound on-ramp. In an hour and fifteen minutes, the rig would exit at Henderson, Louisiana, near the edge of the Atchafalaya River Swamp.

Mia decided to get herself a motel room in Lafayette and wait after she dumped Milt. She was sleepy and needed rest. As she showered, reality and the gravity of the situation she had put herself in dawned on her as she began to calm down. Milt's words replayed in her mind as she dried herself and sat on the edge of the bed. Like a sixteen-pound sledgehammer hitting her between the eyes, Mia cried out to the empty motel room, "My God. What have I done? I can never go see my baby again and never be friends with Lea." She grabbed her cell phone and dialed.

The gruff voice on the other end answered already knowing who was calling asked, "What is it now, Mia?

"We got to get that man out of that trailer before he freezes to death."

"Damnit to hell, can't you make up your mind what you want or what?" the gruff voice answered.

"I don't want to kill that man. I just wanted to scare the hell out of him. That's all I wanted to do."

"Little late for that Baby Girl. That man is probably frozen solid by now. I turned my unit down to thirty below. I'll go check and see if he is still with us. If he is, I'll dump him and drive off and leave him," said the man.

"Would you call me back and let me know either way?" Mia pleaded.

"Yeah, I'll call," answered the irritated man hanging up.

Twenty minutes later Mia received bad news that would forever change her life. Ryan was frozen stiff. The man told her not to come to Henderson. He would take care of everything. He told her that he would not be back for a while because he was heading to the West Coast with a load of fryers out of Mississippi and then planned to run produce to the northeast out of California for while.

Mia had told the man what was going on and about how they were setting up Norris. He would have to handle this just right. Living on the edge all his life, he would handle this matter and walk away laughing to himself. After all, he owed Mia more than he could ever repay.

Depression racked Mia's mind in waves as she sat on the bed and shook her head. Rigors cursed her body as she lamented about losing Sly, Lea, and Milt. This was her family she had betrayed in a self-centered rage against a man who probably had not done anything more than men used to do to her when she was that age. True, it was a sorry bastard that would hit on a young girl, but most girls were taught early to brush it off. Would Lea and Milt ever let her see her baby again? Probably not. Would Lynn ever have anything to do with her again? Never. Lea proved that yesterday afternoon at Amber's shop. Lying down on the bed clad only in her panties, Mia beat the pillow as she wailed on about how sorry she was for everything.

Mercifully, the sandman paid a short visit to Mia. She slept fitfully for thirty-four minutes; then Mia bolted upright in the bed, knowing she must go home and beg forgiveness from Lea, Milt, Lynn, and Amber. She dressed quickly, gathered up her stuff—never once looking back, locked the motel, door leaving the room key on the dresser, and headed toward the house to try to make amends.

She pulled into a convenience store for a cup of coffee, leaving the clerk the change from a five as a tip. Realizing it was at least an hour and forty-five minutes to Oakwood, she gouged the Yukon. Early morning traffic was extra heavy on Interstate 10 between Lafayette and Lake Charles. After being cut off twice in the heavy traffic, Mia hit the steering wheel with her right hand and screamed again into the windshield, "Don't anybody ever stay home any more?"

She had to force herself to stay awake before she got to Lake Charles. She willed herself to keep driving and get home. She stopped for a cold soda trying to force herself awake at her exit to Oakwood. The road to Oakwood was brand-new asphalt overlay, two-lane, smooth as a billiard table with paved shoulders. Mia pushed the Yukon up to seventy-six in a fifty-five miles per hour speed zone and set the cruise control breaking two cardinal safe driving rules: never

ever use cruise control if you are tired and sleepy and above every other rule in the book, do not drive if you are sleepy.

The cold soda lacked enough caffeine to fight back the drowsiness from the lack of sleep. In a long stretch of highway with no traffic, the involuntary sleep reflexes overrode Mia's will power to stay awake as her eyes slowly lost focus and her head dropped slightly. The left front tire eased over the centerline stripe. The slight crown in the center of the road slightly changed the inertia of the heavy SUV as it slewed even more into the opposite lane, overriding the superb suspension system on the Yukon. The air bags were rendered useless as teats on a boar hog as the heavy truck slammed into the reinforced concrete bridge abutment at seventy-six miles per hour driving the engine, transmission, left front wheel, and steering column through the firewall of the engine compartment into the rear seat of the Yukon taking its sleeping driver with it. Mia Comeaux would have been thirty-three in six days.

Lea suggested that they eat before they went home. She was starving and certain that Lynn and Milt were famished as well. Referred to locally as the Greasy Spoon Café, the City Grill on Main Street opened at five-thirty and closed at seven-thirty seven days a week. Todd Mire, nicknamed Toddy, was a second-generation restaurateur. He inherited the City Grill from his dad and mom, and now he and his wife Leona operated the grill. Breakfast and sandwiches were the fare. Toddie had not changed a thing except the coffee-making machine since he took over the café nearly seventeen years ago.

Lynn, Milt, and Lea sat in the back booth, ordering breakfast. Milt and Lynn eat breakfast at the Greasy Spoon frequently, Leona knew what they liked and how they wanted it fixed. Lea ordered a cheese omelet with black coffee. Milt was still mad as hell at Mia and himself. Lea and Lynn listened to his raving but never offered any input. Finally Lea said softly, "Milt, we have to get this behind us and move on. Let's eat and go to the house and shower and go get everybody paid and take a nap. Maybe by then we'll will hear from Amber or maybe even Mia. Okay?"

Toby was not overly alarmed when he discovered that Ryan hadn't made it in last night. Probably found a girl to sleep over with. Toby dressed in cut-off jeans, faded Dallas Cowboy's tee shirt, and leather sandals walked toward the convenience store for a cup of coffee and sausage and cheese croissant. Riding her bike from Paw's to her house, Sly stopped to talk a minute with Toby. Sly was gushing with the news that somebody had called from Nashville yesterday and the day before also. Toby asked who called and Sly admitted that she really didn't know because they never talked to her. Toby assured her that he and Ryan were delighted to know that the recording companies in Nashville responded so quickly. "After all, Sly, they are in the business of finding real talent. You have the talent and looks to make it big-time. But above all of that, I admire your guitar picking. Very few pickers can match your playing ability. No one I have ever seen can sing and play melody like you can. Willie Nelson and Waylon Jennings are exceptions, you understand," said Toby, sincerely complementing Sly.

"I certainly do understand. I practice every day and try hard to be the best I can be."

"You are almost there, Sly. Maybe a couple of years early, but trust me; you are on the brink of something great for yourself. Do you think you can handle being rich and famous?" asked Toby.

"Yeah, as long as I can return to Oakwood and everybody will leave me alone. Sure, I believe I can handle all that," Sly replied.

"When your first album hits the stores and your picture is on every magazine cover and you are doing the big concerts, your life as you know it will be only memories, Sly," said Toby continuing with, "Trust me. I know because I've seen it happen lot of times."

"I am willing to make the sacrifice if Mama and Daddy will let me. If they won't let me start now I'll bide my time and when Mama and Daddy give me to myself, Toby, country music, here I come. I got to go. See you later," said Sly giving Toby the smile that soon would be engraved in every young man's mind in America.

Sly sensed that things weren't right when she got home that morning. Daddy was in a snit like she had never seen him before. Sly asked her Mama what was going on with Daddy. Lea assured her daughter that it was nothing really, only adding more doubt to the teenager's mind.

"You and Daddy didn't have a good time last night? I thought you and Daddy went out with Aunt Mia and Lynn, Mama," said Sly.

"Yes, Sly, but we didn't have a good time. Your Aunt Mia sort of got out of line and that is the end of the story, okay?"

"Yes ma'am," answered Sly, wondering what Aunt Mia could have done to get her daddy in a snit.

After chowing down on his croissant and coffee, Toby walked a few blocks to uptown. Standing on the main street he looked south towards Sam's place. He immediately recognized their rusted out Corolla parked near Sam's. Toby moseyed off down the street knowing he would probably find Ryan at Sam's, shooting the bull with Sam and his waitresses. Sure enough, the Corolla was parked in front of Sam's, but Sam wasn't open yet. Toby checked out the car and found the key in the ignition switch, something neither one seldom ever did. Everything else seemed in order. Ryan's cloth briefcase, cell phone, a tennis racket and three balls, two dirty towels, a pair of flip-flops, and two dirty T-shirts were on the back seat. At least six empty pizza boxes on the back floorboard. Toby shrugged and walked back toward his apartment.

Hardly anyone would speak to him anymore because of what Ryan had been doing to the young girls. Toby could sense the tension in the air when he was around folks who knew who he and Ryan were. Toby had told Ryan that next week was his last in Oakwood. Ryan had agreed that it was time to move on, maybe out to the left coast where folks are a tad more tolerant.

It was early in the morning when Amber called. She was calmed down somewhat but still apprehensive about Mia's double-cross. Lea assured Amber that Mia probably had turned Ryan loose and was playing the mind game with them. "Mia plays rough sometimes, Amber. It's just her way of doing things," said Lea trying to convince Amber and herself everything would turn out okay. Lea was pissing into the wind as far convincing Amber of anything of the sort. This was not Amber's first rodeo. She could sense real trouble for all of them not far down the pike.

Busy as a cranberry merchant, Lea finished up her payroll and settlement checks for their owner-operators, and logging crew realizing that she was beyond tired and sleepy. Milt had gone out to the shop to deliver the checks to the loggers and drivers. Lea deposited the owner-operators checks by direct deposit. Into her fourth cup of coffee and some aspirin for her nagging headache, she sat back in her office chair going over the events of the past week or so. What she thought was going to be a huge wedding with Mia and Lynn had gone south. Discovering Sly's singing talent was overwhelming. The mess they had gotten themselves into was discouraging and would probably get them all into serious trouble. Sipping her coffee and reflecting on all her problems, Lea, thinking about last night with Lynn said to herself, "It's all gonna work out. I just know it will."

The ringing of the telephone on her desk finally jarred her back into reality. Lea answered the phone noting on the caller ID that it was the sheriff's office. "Lea, this is Alden. I'm afraid I have some bad news, Hon."

"What's the matter, Sheriff Malone?" asked Lea picking up on the stress in his voice.

"It's Mia, Lea. She was killed in a wreck about an hour ago about twelve miles south of town," answered the sheriff his voice breaking waiting for Lea to answer him.

"Please tell me you may be mistaken. Please don't let it be her," sobbed Lea.

"I'm so sorry but I also called to ask a favor from you or Milt. One of you need to positively identify the body. I could do it but the rules won't let me. Her mama broke down when we told her, and she is in the emergency room at Lake Charles. Her step dad is in a nursing home. I guess it boils down to you since your daddy and mama are out of town, baby."

"I'll get Milt to come. I want to remember her like she was the last time I saw her."

"That'll be just fine. They haven't got her body out of the truck yet. It's the worst wreck I've seen in a long time," said the sheriff as he continued, "I'm so sorry Lea. I know you were like sisters. I offer my sincere condolences."

Lea sat numbed at the heart rendering news. Finally she called Milt and told him to come to the house. "I have some bad news. I want you home now," sobbed Lea into the phone.

Milt was home in minutes. Lea met him at the door and hugged him, crying her heart out. Sly was in her room playing music, unaware of the news of Mia's wreck. Milt finally took her face in his hands and asked, "What's the matter. Tell me, baby. What's the matter?"

"It's Mia, Milt. Mia is dead. She was killed in car wreck on the way home."

"Where did it happen?"

"Sheriff Malone called and told me about it. He said it happened twelve miles south of town about an hour ago."

"What happened?

"He didn't go into all of that. He wants one of us to come and identify the body. I told him you would. I don't want to see her all mangled up and remember her that way. Will you do that for me?"

"Yeah, I'll go right now and see what I can do."

"Before you go I want you to be here with me when I tell Sly," said Lea still crying as she went to get Sly.

Sly handled it pretty good for a teenager. She cried because her Mamma and Daddy were so upset. She went to her room to grieve for her Aunt Mia in private. She had been sort of miffed at Aunt Mia lately because Mia didn't want her to pursue a country music singing career.

Chapter 12

While Mia lay a corpse at the funeral home in Oakwood, the story about the man frozen to death and dumped at the Butte Larose rest area on I-10 captured local headline news. Now, the only person who Lynn, Lea, Amber, and Milt knew for sure what happened was dead and the identity of her accomplice unknown. Lynn and Amber stood outside the funeral home the night of Mia's wake and talked about it among themselves. Lynn said since Mia was dead, probably the only chance of the law connecting Ryan's death to them was that if Ryan had told his partner Toby where he was going the night he came to his place to see Anna. Amber told Lynn that the word on the street was that Toby had left town. Amber suggested to Lynn that they should ride by Toby's place and see if his car was still there.

"I have to find out something to give Lea some peace of mind," remarked Lynn.

"You gotta be real careful about what you ask and who you ask, Lynn. Never know who's gonna stab you in the back," answered Amber, "What are your plans now that Mia is gone, if I might be so bold to ask?" asked Amber.

"Don't know yet. I'm gonna take a few days off and try to get my head straight and then I don't know. Why?" answered Lynn.

"Well, let me say this, Mia helped me when I come back home. She helped me get my shop and my life back on track. I liked Mia until night before last when she lost it. Somehow, I just can't make myself believe she really wanted to kill Ryan. For some odd reason, don't ask me why though, I think she just wanted to punish him a little more than we did and something went bad wrong. You know what I'm trying to say, Lynn, Mia wanted to be just a little more redneck or bronckey than the rest of us," remarked Amber, firing off a cigarette hoping to chase away the mosquitoes with the smoke.

"I don't guess we'll ever know for sure but I would certainly like to believe what you said and just let her rest in peace," said Lynn closing the subject. "I think I'm gonna ride by Toby's place and see if his car is still there. You want to ride with me?"

"Sure. Why not? Pick me up at Sam's and we'll check out ole Toby. That boy may know too much for his own good if you know what I mean," said Amber as she left to find her car in the parking lot.

Lynn watched Amber as she walked away for a moment. He had never seen Amber all fixed up and wearing a dress in his entire life. She was looking fine. Amber knew he was checking her out. A pang of guilt gored him as he stood in front of the funeral home where his lady friend lay a corpse and lusted after Amber as he watched her walk to her car.

Lynn picked up Amber and they headed towards Toby's apartment. Sure enough, the street talk was correct unless he was working at the radio station tonight. His car wasn't parked at the apartment complex. A trip by the radio station drew a blank. They decided to cruise around town looking for the car. After nearly a half-hour of riding, looking, and talking, Lynn asked Amber if she was hungry. They decided on a burger and sat in the pickup and ate. Lynn's pickup windows were tinted and it would be hard for someone to see Amber riding around with Lynn. As they ate, Amber broached the subject of Toby again.

Lynn explained that Toby and Ryan worked as a team. Since Ryan was gone, maybe he had pulled stakes and left town. Amber pulled her phone out and called the radio station's number by memory because the last four digits of the number were the stations call letters. The phone rang ten times at least before some goofy-ass boy answered. Amber inquired about how to reach Toby. The goof ball, trying his dumb ass best to be professional, hesitated with the answers. Amber turned up the hot talk and finally flirted an answer out of him after she promised to drink a soda with him at Sam's later.

"Where on earth do these radio stations find these weirdoes, Lynn? That little jerk-off couldn't even carry on a conversation.

Started every sentence with "like." But he did say that Toby has drug up. Left for California late this afternoon. You know, Lynn, that Toby guy is a nice-looking man. I cut his hair a couple of times. He asked me out as a matter of fact. I was seriously considering dating him until I found out he was staying with the sicko."

"To hell you say! Mia went out with him just before we got together. That boy really gets around, don't he?"

"Yeah. He told me that he liked women a little older than himself. Boy, that sucker was full of hisself."

"By the way, where's Norris at tonight?"

"He come the funeral home as soon as they opened at four o'clock. Said he had to go see about his mama in the hospital. She had a gallstone operation that ain't turning out too good. You know his mama and daddy takes care of that boy of his while he's on the road. Got a mobile home in his yard."

"You and Norris getting serious or something?"

"It's this way, Lynn. I like Norris. He's a good old boy if he don't talk about that lush ex-wife of his. I done told him I ain't listening to all that shit about her. I done been stung too many times to let my feelings get too carried away with any man, if that will answer your question."

"Would you consider going out with me?" asked Lynn being a little bit cocky but serious enough for Amber to ponder the question a minute before she answered.

"You damned right I would. It really would look better if we waited a while though. Whatcha think?"

"Bullshit. I don't have to wait no year before I date another woman, Amber. Mia ain't my wife."

"I know all that, big boy," said Amber laughing and patting his thigh. "About a week or two oughta be long enough if you can wait that long. What about you and Lea? You going to still slip around and see her?"

"Naw, we both got what we missed in high school, and she is still very much in love with Milt."

"That don't mean crap. Some women like more than one man just like some men like to slip around on their wives or girlfriends. She'll be back for more if you were any good. Trust me. Mia told me all about your credentials."

"You are full of it, girl," answered Lynn.

"This dress is giving me a fit. Too long to start with," said Amber kicking off her shoes, raising up, and pulling the hemline all the way up to her hips, "I'm a jeans and shorts gal. Don't wear dresses much. Don't mind if I get comfortable do you, Lynn?"

"Not at all. I like the scenery," said Lynn admiring her long slender legs as dark as Anna's.

Amber turned, leaning her back on the door of the pickup and stretched her legs out across the seat laying her feet on Lynn's right thigh as she looked over the top of her fountain drink sucking on the straw and smiling. "You said you liked the scenery. While you're sightseeing I'm going to get comfortable," said Amber licking her lips as she watched Lynn's reaction to her boldness. Her toes, Lynn noticed, were extraordinarily long and slender. Amber's toenails were pedicured to perfection. Lynn's hand rubbed Amber's ankles and played with her toes. Not ticklish, his playing with her toes excessively made Amber wonder if Lynn was a toe sucker. If he didn't stop, this self- imposed waiting period would definitely have to be waived. His big hand ventured up to the calves of her long legs, caressing them as they tried to make small talk. Amber dug her heel into his crotch ever so easy, trying to see if he was aroused. Lynn leaned toward Amber as he worked his way up her legs with both hands. Amber's feet now reached the inside of his left thigh. As she gently felt his crotch with the ball of her foot, she now knew why Lea and Mia were crazy for this man.

The ringing telephone stopped Amber and Lynn from seducing each other. Anna called to tell Lynn that his horses were out and she needed him to come home and help get them back in the pasture. Lynn took Amber back to get her car and promised to call her soon.

Hot, muggy winds blew in from the Gulf as the funeral procession stopped at the graveyard. Mia's last ride was to a small graveyard five miles out of Oakwood. All of her mother's family was interred in this small cemetery beside this small Methodist church. Mia's funeral services were at the funeral home in Oakwood. The family was expecting ten times the number of people that the small country church could seat, they weren't disappointed. Mia's wake and funeral were the largest in anyone's memory ever held in Oakwood. So many people came to pay their last respects that it was standing room only outside on the lawn of the funeral home. Sue and Roger Hart, Mia's bosses, and Lea's mom and dad took over the funeral arrangements for Mia's mother. Sue and Roger gave Mia the head start in style and dignity.

Mia's grieving mom could not bring herself to try to settle Mia's estate. It was assumed that Mia's mom would inherit everything. The district judge appointed Roger Hart administrator of Mia's estate to quickly settle her affairs and pay the funeral home and other bills. Roger knew that Mia was very well off indeed. She had invested wisely in property and the stock market. Her checking account balance was ten times what it should have been. Roger and Sue were going through her personal papers at her house when the man at the bank called and informed Roger that Mia had a safety deposit box and would open it for him if he brought the key. The key was located and Roger and Sue showed up at the local bank to retrieve the contents of Mia's safety deposit box.

To the astonishment of Sue and Roger as well as everyone that knew her, Mia recently had a will drawn by a lawyer friend in Beaumont as a favor to her after they were involved in a huge land-swapping deal for an oil company. The preamble letter attached to the sealed brown envelope stated that if Roger outlived Mia, he was to be named the executor of her estate. Roger took the preamble letter and unopened brown envelope to the district judge to set up a reading of Mia's will.

The next morning the judge's office notified Lea to bring Sly to the judges office indicating that Sly was a benefactor named in Mia's will. Lea wondered what she left Sly.

At ten sharp, the district judge walked into a small courtroom set up for these purposes and announced that he would read Mia's last will and testament. He said he had read it and found it to be in good order and called the lawyer in Beaumont who wrote it for her. Mia left three hundred thousand dollars to her mother, along with a nice house that she had remodeled and was renting. To her real dad, thought to be somewhere in Mississippi, Mia bequeathed three hundred thousand dollars and one nice rent property in Orange, Texas. To her stepsiblings she left not a single dollar.

Lea sat there listening, never realizing before now much money Mia had made, saved, and invested until the judge started giving her estate away. Lea realized that not once had Mia ever mentioned her wealth or the will. First, a trust fund was already set up for Sly's college education with enough money in it to become a doctor if Sly was so inclined. Lastly, Sly inherited everything else Mia owned: her home, land, rent properties, stock portfolio, checking account, and Mia's jewelry—everything. When the counting was done Sly walked out of the courthouse a wealthy teenage girl. Roger was named trustee of the estate until Sly became of majority age, which was just fine because Sly was his only grandchild. The judge commented that Mia was an exceptionally good businessperson to accumulate assets in that range at a young age.

This frozen man case was getting on the Lafayette Parish district attorney's last nerve with every major news network shoving a video camera and mike in his face every time he showed his face in public, asking questions that he couldn't answer. An excellent lawyer and outstanding and popular DA, Leonce Lemoyne was completely forthcoming with the press. He simply told them that right now they knew as much as he did. However, the state police had volunteered their services to move the investigation to a higher level, meaning that the governor said, "Find the person who did this horrific crime and find him before the trail gets cold." The governor was also being constantly harassed by the media along with the sheriff of Lafayette Parish. Every politician loves a TV camera except when asked the hard questions that can't be answered. Leonce didn't like being put on the spot without answers.

The receptionist in the DA's office put Dr. Lance Goudeaux, Lafayette Parish coroner, through to Leonce Lemoyne, the district attorney for Lafayette Parish, immediately. Dr. Goudeaux stated that the DA, the sheriff, Sergeant Cecil Bell, and himself needed to meet and discuss the Frappé Monsieur case in detail. Dr. Goudeaux loved mysteries and considered himself a present day Sherlock Holmes. The good doctor's perception in fact was far greater than the average person, the DA knew he was a man who could tie facts and hunches together and agreed to set up a meeting. Dr. Goudeaux had helped him and the sheriff several times before. The sheriff thought he was psychic. Like any real Cajun invitation, Dr. Goudeaux told Leonce to arrange the meeting, tonight if possible, and he would fix supper for everyone. Loving company and parties Dr. Goudeaux insisted that everyone bring their family. The DA's receptionist thought Dr. Goudeaux could walk on water. He had delivered all three of her children.

Forgoing prior dinner plans, Leonce decided that maybe they could come up with something that may have been overlooked in their investigation. Leonce and his secretary quickly arranged for all parties and their families to be at Dr. Lance's at seven-thirty.

Mosquito lamps burning on the bamboo stands strategically placed around the patio at Dr. Goudeaux's palatial home near Broussard were doing a creditable job keeping the insects at bay. Noisy but not boisterous children played in and around the swimming pool as the adults watched and talked on the patio. Cajuns know the art of conversation and partying. Dr. Goudeaux and his wife Alicia were always gracious hosts to a fault, and enjoyed entertaining at their home. Dr. Goudeaux was grilling steaks for the grown-ups and burgers for the children. Sergeant Bell's teenage son and the sheriff's teen-age daughter had opted for a steak not wanting to lumped into the children-hamburger category..

After one of best meals any of the guests had eaten in recent memory, Dr. Goudeaux indicated that the men retire to the den to discuss the frozen man. His wife remarked to the other women after the men went inside that this frozen man (frappé monsieur thing) had bothered Lance more than anything she could ever remember.

Leonce opened with why this case needed to be solved quickly, indicating that the news media coverage could ruin some careers if some answers didn't show up soon. Everyone nodded in agreement. Leonce asked Sergeant Bell if he brought the tape of all the interviews he did the night of the investigation. Sergeant Bell pulled a copy of the original from his shirt pocket, indicating he had complied with the DA's request.

Dr. Goudeaux took the tape and opened the doors of a huge home-entertainment system cabinet wherein a superb tape deck swallowed the tape as the doctor inserted it into the machine. Dr. Goudeaux made a few adjustments as the machine began to play the interviews.

Everyone but the coroner had heard the tape twenty or more times. As the tape played, Dr. Goudeaux listened intently as the other three men drifted into hushed conversation.

Dr. Goudeaux turned and with his right hand swiped the clam-it-up sign and backed the tape up and started it again, turning the volume louder. He stepped over to a cabinet and retrieved a box of fine imported cigars and passed the box to his guests. Having had a hell of a time getting off the cigarette habit, Sergeant Bell reluctantly took one as well as the sheriff and the DA. The host lit his cigar and passed the lighter to his guests as he laughingly said, "I know all of you have listened to this tape a thousand times. I've never did hear it yet, me," speaking in the Cajun-English dialect used by most Cajuns when conversing informally among friends. The coroner stood as he listened intently to the tape. Throwing up both hands, the coroner stopped the tape again and rewound it to listen to the interview with the second truck driver that Sergeant Bell interviewed. As he started the tape again he picked up a note pad and pen from the side table by his recliner and started making notes. His guests through thick cigar smoke watched him scribble.

Finally, after two more rewinds, Dr. Goudeaux asks Sergeant Bell to carefully try to remember everything about this man that he could. His mannerisms, his attitude, anything out of the ordinary.

Sergeant Bell related his interview to his peers as carefully and accurately as he remembered, concluding that Raymond Cloyd was never considered a suspect at all. In fact he was helpful and straightforward with all his answers.

"Did you happen to talk to Cloyd off the tape, Cecil? Like asking some personal questions?" asked Dr. Goudeaux.

"No. Everything is on the tape," answered Cecil not being completely forthcoming with the coroner resenting the fact that Dr. Goudeaux was attempting to build a case against Raymond Cloyd.

"Several questions have surfaced about this Cloyd guy that bother me. I had a few beers that night but he seemed just a little bit too unconcerned about the whole affair. It's not a common thing to find a man frozen to death around here, if you know what I mean. This ain't Alaska," said the coroner.

"You got that shot right, Doc," Leonce remarked. "Why does this guy have your suspicion up is what I'd like to know?"

"Three or four things really, Leonce. First, he examines the body. I didn't notice the corpse's fingernails and fingers. He did. Mr. Cloyd stated that the cuts on the victim jaw, lower lip, ear, and leg were the results of a beating. I'm almost positive that a dog inflicted those wounds, especially the cuts on the victim's leg and jaw. He said they dumped his dead ass out of the horse blanket. How could Cloyd know that the man and two women were dumping a dead body?" asked Dr. Goudeaux looking at each man, beaming his know-it-all smile.

"How I missed that is beyond me," said the sheriff. "This does put the Cloyd man in a different light so to speak, huh, Cecil?"

Careful not to get stampeded into a witch-hunt, Cecil replied, "Raymond Cloyd knew that the object was a corpse when I taped the interview. What are your other points, Doc?"

Up and pacing the floor, Dr. Goudeaux checked his notes, took a long drag on his cigar, and looked at each of his guests momentarily as he exhaled the aromatic cigar smoke, carefully choosing his words. "We need to be looking for a missing pedophile. We can start from here back tracking and tie this Cloyd man to this murder. I'm certain that is the answer to this mystery," replied Dr. Goudeaux looking at the ceiling fan waiting to be regaled with questions.

After a minute of silence, Cecil commented, "Cloyd did refer to the fact that it was a stretch but the frappé monsieur could have been a child molester."

"Exactly!" exclaimed Dr. Goudeaux, "Why on earth would Cloyd mention a child molester unless he was aware of the fact that indeed the man was pedophilic before he was murdered?"

"You suggesting to us that Cloyd interjected his innuendoes in his clever statement to Cecil, never thinking someone would figure him out?" asked Leonce.

"Hell yeah, bro. The probability of someone else even thinking about a pedophile, much less offering the child molestation angle into a statement to an officer, is astronomical at this point. What I am saying is that this bastard is rattling the investigators' cages and laughing at them," said the coroner shaking his head assuring himself that he was right.

"Accusing the only eyewitness to this crime is way out in left field, even for you, Doc," cut in Cecil.

Undaunted by Cecil's remark, Dr. Goudeaux shot back, "The facts are there. Get your head out of your drawers and think. This man was playing you like a drum. I know you don't like having this shit slung in your face, bro, but I'd bet my left testicle that I'm right. Whatcha think, Leonce?"

"I have to say that your theory is the best I've heard yet," answered Leonce.

"I say we start looking for a missing child molester, Cecil. If we find one I'm betting the frappé monsieur will be him. We can keep what we discussed among us. It won't be hard to find out all about this man once we identify him. That gives us two ends to work from. Surely we ought to know who the frozen man is by tomorrow or the next day," said Sheriff John Miller.

John Miller, like Alden Malone, had been sheriff of Lafayette Parish a long time. Grown men and women with families had never known another sheriff in Lafayette Parish. In all southern parishes local politics is always in the forefront. Every election someone always ran against John Miller. The opponent always lost. John never tired of politicking. He liked being sheriff. Speaking French fluently, John communicated well with the native-born Cajun people in Lafayette Parish as well as the huge influx of oilfield people who migrated to his parish from elsewhere. Above all else, John was a graduate of LSU law school. Passed the bar exam and never practiced law. He was in the Secret Service for ten years in Washington D. C. Returning home at the age of thirty-three, he was elected sheriff. John Miller's career as sheriff spanned thirty-one years of public service. A fishing buddy of the sitting governor, John had lots of political clout.

"Cloyd is from Mississippi. If he hauled that man to the Butte Larose exit they ain't no telling where the frozen man is from. Talking about a needle in the haystack, this is even worse, we don't even know where the damned haystack is." said Cecil, miffed at the others for thinking that Cloyd was the perpetrator.

"We will start looking tonight and continue until we have exhausted all resources. Right sheriff?" said Leonce.

"Absolutely. I'm leaving shortly for the office and have the dispatcher and detectives start the search immediately. Tomorrow I will personally call around to the other parishes in south Louisiana and make some inquiries," announced the High Sheriff.

"What about you, Cecil?" asked Leonce.

"I will start looking. I will call Baton Rouge and try to get some more investigators over here to help out," answered Cecil getting to his feet. Leonce also got up indicating it was time to gather up their families and head to the house.

"Cecil, no hard feelings?" asked Dr. Goudeaux sincerely as he shook Cecil's hand.

"No. Maybe this time I trusted my instinct more than the facts. See you later. Thanks for the great food and inviting my family," said Cecil as walked out on the patio to gather his family.

Chapter 13

True to his word, Sheriff John Miller stopped by his office on the way home to begin the search for a missing child molester, a missing child that might have been molested, and any reports of charges of child molestation. The officers at the sheriff's office knew that this had something to do with the frozen man case, but not a single officer questioned the sheriff about this strange turn of the investigation. Reports were already filtering in before the sheriff went home. His orders were to print out every report and have them all on his desk when he returned in the morning.

At seven-thirty, the following morning one hundred and four recent reports of child molestation lay on his desk from the Gulf Coast region alone. The sheriff looked at these as he wondered how many were from his parish. He found out later that four were from his parish, two involving the clergy. John was about to walk out of office to the coffeepot and jaw with his deputies, a morning ritual that started the first day he was in office, when he noticed he had e-mail. He punched up his e-mail on his computer. One message perked his interest. It simply stated, "Call me today. Alden Malone." Wondering if this concerned their next sheriff association meeting, John almost let Alden's e-mail note slide. He decided to call Alden and shoot the bull for a few minutes after he went to the coffeepot.

John made the coffeepot bull session seven mornings a week, even coming to the office for a while on the weekends just to stay on top of everything going on in his parish. If his officers knew any news or just gossip it was informally aired in these few minutes each morning. With the door to the breakroom closed, each deputy was cautioned never to discuss anything or comments made herein with the public, not even family. A lot of talk about the solution of the Frappé Monsieur case floated around the break room. John Miller listened carefully to each person's speculation about the frozen man case. John revealed that his office was taking a different approach to the investigation of the case. He told the reporters in the hall that he expected to identify the frozen man by tomorrow. At ten after eight, John sits down at his desk again asking his secretary to call Alden Malone. Alden like himself had been sheriff a long time. The sheriff's secretary called to say she had Sheriff Alden Malone on line four, his private line.

After exchanging the usual pleasantries, Sheriff Alden asked, "I heard you are looking for a missing child molester."

"That's right, Alden. I'm going about this Frappé Monsieur case sort of in a backwards way trying to find out who da hell dis guy is and above all who iced him," the Lafayette Parish High Sheriff chuckled. "Man, we ain't got a damn clue bout dis dude, Alden. You hear me, man?"

"Well, I just might be able to help you out there a little bit, ole partner. A while back two young men moved down here to Oakwood and went to work for the local radio station. Their names are Ryan Roberts and Toby Nichols. Ryan Roberts is the man's radio show name. His real name is Sanford L. Brooks. He and Nichols are both twenty-seven. Both of them are from Greeley, Colorado, area. I checked all this out yesterday. Now here is the kicker, John. This Ryan boy comes up missing a few days ago and his partner, Toby has done up and left town the evening of Mia Comeaux's wake two days ago.

"Yeah, I done read about dat girl in da paper. I met her at a party in Lake Charles a couple months ago. Talk about pretty and smart; man, that girl had it all. I'm so sorry to hear about her death, Alden. Did you know her very good?" interrupted John.

"Aw man, did I ever. I watched that girl grown up. That woman caused a car wreck over here a while back just walking down da street. This man was watching her rear end and not the road—rear-ended another car," said Alden laughing, "Yeah John, Mia will be sadly missed. She put lotta smiles on men's faces. I'll tell you what, man. That woman done made herself helluva lot of money selling real estate."

"Yeah. I know. Man, she was something else. Uh—about them radio station boys you was ah fixing to tell about when I interrupted to talk about a pretty woman. What's going down over dare with dem dudes, Alden?" asked John.

"Well, like I said, it seems that Ryan would fool these young girls over to his apartment then have his way with them. No one filed a complaint against him, but I have heard that he nailed at least four girls from 'round here, all under fifteen. You know, John, folks around here don't take to this kind of crap. I'm not pushing anything yet until I have a complaint. But I can get you something to match up his DNA if you want to try to match your man up with Ryan Roberts. To tell you truth, John, if I knew that child molesting Ryan Roberts was indeed the Frappé Monsieur and nobody complained or seen it happen I would have never opened a serious investigation. That's how I feel 'bout it myself."

Sheriff John Miller listened carefully to his old friend in Oakwood as he jotted down names and places on his yellow legal pad. "Yeah, Alden I feel da same way, but dis shit is in my ballpark and I'm under big time pressure to find some answers and lock somebody's ass up. They done run the frozen man's DNA. Can you send Dr. Jude John something at the crime lab in Baton Rouge? This frozen guy is about twenty-seven according to my information, Alden, I do thank you for all this information and I'll check these two guys out. You don't have any hunches or suspects who might have made this Ryan Roberts disappear do you, Alden?" asked John easing off on his Cajun dialect some.

"Can't help you there. Ain't nobody filed a missing persons report yet," lied the Oakwood sheriff. "I'm gonna call the Crime Lab for you and get them to go ahead and put the crime lab folks in the helicopter and send them on over here for you. Be lot quicker that way."

"Man, I owe you big-time. Let me know if anything else comes up over there that might concern this matter. Alden, thanks and I'll see you at the association meeting," said John Miller hanging up the phone, his brow knitted in deep thought.

Alden Malone knew just about everything that happened in Adams Parish. Alden was the first law officer figure out the identity of the Frappé Monsieur. He wanted all the media commotion to stay in Lafayette, keeping his hunch to himself. He knew who had reefer trailers in Oakwood, who was missing, and who had teenage daughters. He smiled to himself thinking, "Some things folks just don't need to know."

John Miller sat at his desk pondering the information that Alden had just laid on him. Why would Alden contact me to pass on street gossip? Was ole Alden covering up something for somebody over in Adams Parish? His secretary brought him a cup of coffee and asked if he had any leads on the iceman case yet. John indicated that she take a seat. The lady who sat before him had helped him get elected many years ago and was the first person he hired after he took office. John appointed a chief deputy but everyone knew who the boss was when John wasn't there. He told her exactly what Alden had told him and then asked her take on the information. She thought about what he had told her for a minute. She advised her boss to go with what he had and let the chips fall where they may.

John picked up the phone to send the State Police to Ryan's Oakwood apartment. Unknown to John, the state police had initiated their own investigation of Ryan Roberts as soon as Alden Malone called and introduced Ryan as a candidate for the Frappé Monsieur before the chopper lifted off from Baton Rouge for Oakwood.

Toby, sweating his ass off in New Mexico, stopped and called Ryan's cell phone once more. No answer. Toby was in a panic, almost certain that the man found frozen was his friend and partner. How long would it be before the authorities found him and made him tell all about Ryan? They would probably accuse him of rape in Louisiana just so they could extradite him and charge him with something. Ryan never told him where he was going that night. He wondered if Ryan had talked Sly into meeting him somewhere and gotten caught. Ryan had sure messed up their plans to go big time with Sly. Toby was pissed off at Ryan, never once giving thought of grieving for his friend.

Getting rid of the old Corolla was his first priority. He sold the car, and then hitchhiked to Prescott, Arizona. He landed a job on the first interview with a mid-sized radio station. He assumed his deceased father's name and social security number. Maybe he would be safe for a few weeks. Then he planned to move on to California. In hours the law would be looking for him with a vengeance.

Toby had left all of Ryan's stuff in the apartment in case he showed up later. Toby knew when Ryan came up missing he would be in serious trouble if and when Ryan was found dead. When the State Police showed up to get DNA samples they gathered up Ryan's comb, toothbrush, and razor along with several other items and left for Baton Rouge. In two hours, Dr. Jude John was running a DNA match.

Tests results were conclusive. The frozen man's real name was Sanford L. Brooks, a.k.a. Ryan Roberts from Greeley, Colorado. John Miller and Alden Malone were the first to know that the frozen man was indeed Ryan. John Miller admitted that the help from Dr. Lance Goudeau helped them get started looking in the right places.

Sergeant Cecil Bell upon hearing the news knew his career could be in jeopardy if he didn't move quickly to apprehend Raymond Cloyd. Dr. Goudeau's assessment of Cloyd had to be true. He called his boss in Baton Rouge and asked if he could be assigned to the investigation unit until Cloyd was apprehended. After a long heated discussion, his boss finally relented and moved him into the investigation unit temporarily. Cecil copied everything in the file on the frozen man case before he left headquarters and took it home with him.

All he could remember about Cloyd was that he was a big guy with a nice beard, clean cut, wore a black cowboy hat, was an owner-operator, and said that he lived in Brandon, Mississippi. He found Cloyd's business card that he had given him the night that the frozen man was found and called the cell phone. Cecil was told that the phone was no longer in service and wasn't listed in Cloyd's name.

With a few calls Cecil found that the cell phone was listed to Katy Kay in Mauriceville, Texas. Cecil called the Orange County sheriff's office asking if they knew Katy Kay and if she was listed in the telephone book.

Yes, she was listed and yes, they knew her quite well. Katy was on the high end of forty, still good-looking, and living in a mobile home in Mauriceville. She had been a cocktail waitress, convenience store clerk, fast-food store manager, a truckstop waitress, a rehabilitated druggie, never arrested, single, no children, and all around likeable woman. The deputy informed Cecil that a couple of years back she enrolled in a truck driving school. After graduation, she'd hooked up with a guy pulling a reefer trailer. When not on the road the trucker lives with her. Cecil asks, "In other words, is she running double cross country with this guy?"

"Yes. They are gone most of the time. I live on the same street as Katy in Mauriceville. She and her man friend are sometimes gone for two or three weeks at a time. My nephew mows the yard and keeps an eye on everything while they are on the road," volunteered the deputy.

Cecil explained that he needed to talk to both of them urgently. Would they send a deputy to see if they were home and hold them until he got there? Readily agreeing to help Cecil, the deputy got Cecil's phone number and dispatched a patrol car to Katy's place.

Fifteen minutes later Cecil's call is returned. Katy isn't home, but the deputy had called around and found out her man friend's name was Raymond Cloyd. Cecil thanked the deputy and walked outside on his patio, thinking about his next move. The late August humidity and heat in Lafayette were stifling. Sipping his coffee, not wanting to mow his yard today, Cecil recalled the deputy's words about Katy. Cecil wondered if she was in the sleeper cab when he was interviewing him. He'd never asked Cloyd if he was driving solo.

Cecil phoned Sheriff Miller to update him on his investigation. Sheriff Miller told Cecil to get in touch with Sheriff Alden Malone over in Adams Parish and ask about Cloyd and Kay. Mauriceville was just over the Louisiana line from Oakwood. He might can help you out in your investigation. Cecil's boss called as soon as Cecil hung up. He informed Cecil that if he had not found and arrested Raymond Cloyd by noon tomorrow, an APB would definitely be issued nationwide and the FBI would probably become involved and take over the investigation. He told Cecil that was all the time he could buy for him and hung up.

With the Louisiana State Police now aware of the possibility of Cloyd's involvement in Ryan's murder, the search began in earnest for Cloyd and Kay. An owner-operator could disappear for weeks if he wanted and work every day. Most owner- operators that run the West Coast operate on an in and out schedule that stays fairly stable timewise. The backhauls are usually loaded close to the drop. The drops are usually regular customers. Gypsy operators go where their brokers send them. If Cloyd was a gypsy-type operator, finding him quickly could pose a problem unless the authorities could be lucky enough to find out if Cloyd used the same broker all the time. Cecil got permission to get a record of all the calls made on Kay's home phone and her new cell phone. An Orange County judge quickly signed the orders for Katy Kay's telephone records to be faxed immediately to the State Police in Baton Rouge. In turn, Baton Rouge headquarters faxed the records to Cecil in Lafayette.

Cecil was in the office when the fax machine spit the records out. Cecil, with the help of some other troopers, quickly ascertained that Cloyd frequently used a broker in Houston. Calling the broker, Cecil found out that Cloyd did indeed pull a lot of loads through this agent. During the course of the conversation Cecil remarked that Cloyd did have a nice truck and reefer unit to work with. "That unit does not belong to Raymond Cloyd. He drives it like an owner-operator, but that unit belongs to Mia Comeaux. Her business address is in Beaumont. The titles and insurance on the tractor and trailer are in her name. I'm looking at copies of her paperwork as I speak," said the broker with the finality of the words "from whence he came" at a graveside. "I've never met the woman; however, I have spoken to her on occasion on the phone. She seems to be an astute businessperson."

"Do you know what the relationship is between Cloyd and Ms. Comeaux?" asked Cecil, hanging on breathless to every word the Houston broker spoke.

"I have not the slightest idea. The paperwork stays in good order, and Mr. Cloyd's CDL is in perfect order with no violations the last time I ran a check. I wish every trucker that I brokered was like Cloyd. He picks up his loads on time and he makes his drops on time. He never asks for advances on the load, and the settlement checks are wired to a bank in Beaumont," answered the broker.

"Are you his exclusive agent, or does he use other brokers?" asked Cecil.

"I'm sure he uses other brokers. All owner-operators use more than one broker. I specialize in reefer loads. I can load my clients with good paying loads to the left coast and reload them with produce back into this area. I send a lot of catfish, seafood, and processed chickens

151

out there. To answer your question: no, not exclusively," replied the broker.

"Is Mr. Cloyd on a run for you?"

"Yes, as a matter of fact, he called earlier. His drop is in Lake Charles at seven this evening. He pulled what we call a short turn. Cloyd took a load of chickens down to McAllen and backhauled South Texas watermelons," said the broker.

"Could you give me the address of the drop?" asked Cecil."

The broker gave Cecil the address of the drop. Cecil thanked the man and hung up.

Cecil decided to drive over to the Sheriff's office and talk to the Sheriff. Updating the Sheriff on his investigation, John again told Cecil, "After you take Cloyd and Kay out of that truck this afternoon, get in touch with Sheriff Alden Malone over in Adams Parish, or better yet take a ride over there and ask Alden all about Cloyd and this Kay woman.

"Okay, but I have to find out about another person involved with Cloyd," said Cecil.

"What's dis shit? Man, don't tell me you done found more peoples to look for, Cecil?"

"Yeah, 'fraid so. That big truck belongs to a Mia Comeaux. She lists her business address as Beaumont, according to the broker I spoke with. She lives at Oakwood over in Adams Parish. I have checked that out already."

"Man, don't come up in here playing dat shit with me, bro," snarled John Miller, jumping to his feet. "You don't know what da hell you talking 'bout now, for sure."

"Whatcha mean by that?" asked Cecil now completely puzzled over John's reaction to the mention of the Comeaux lady's name.

"I knew that woman. She was killed in a car wreck and buried just two days ago. Dat woman ain't involved in no damn trucking, Cecil. She was the biggest real-estate agent on the Gulf Coast. This Comeaux woman lived at Oakwood over in Adams parish that is for shore," protested John Miller loud and clear.

"The man said he was looking at her truck paper work file as we talked. He don't know about any relationship between Ms. Comeaux and Cloyd. I asked."

"Dis is bullshit, Cecil. Why in the world would dat beautiful woman be involved in the trucking business as much money as she done made selling real-estate?" asked John continuing, "Wait a minute. Dat being the case, dat slick ass Alden Malone knows a helluva lot more 'bout this than he told me dis morning, bro."

"Whatcha mean?"

"Alden Malone e-mailed me first thing this morning to call him. I called. He told me that the Comeaux girl lived over there in Oakwood. Then he tells me about this Ryan What's-his-name done come up missing and him being a molester. Truly, he done identified the Frappé Monsieur, but I knowed that boy was holding back on me. I just felt it while we talked."

"I see now where you coming from. Ryan and Ms. Comeaux are from Oakwood but Cloyd had a Mississippi CDL."

"That don't mean shit. Dem CDL's last four years, don't they? He don't really have to get another one till that one expires? Right?"

"Yeah, but they supposed to get one in the state of their residence."

Now calmed down considerably, John Miller was pacing his office floor. Suddenly he turned to Cecil with a smirky smile, announcing, "Bro, am I glad you come by here to pass a good talk."

"I just wanted to get your take on this case, John. I didn't come in here to pull your chain."

"Dat's what I'm saying. Dis is all clear now, Cecil. We're fixing to move this ball game over to Adams Parish. I knew that Alden wasn't leveling with me this morning. If you are investigating this case, you better run to the house and pack a suitcase. You are going to be in Adams Parish a few days," said the Lafayette Parish Sheriff reverting to his business accent leaving the rich Cajun dialect to be used only with his close friends as he walked to the door with Cecil and bid him good luck.

After Cecil left the office John asked his secretary to get Alden Malone on the telephone again. In minutes she had Alden on the phone. John passed the pleasantries. Alden returned them in kind. John asked, "Alden, you remember us talking about the Comeaux girl this morning?"

"Yeah, I do, John. What about her?"

"Was dat girl in the trucking business? Like, ah, how you call dem refrigerator trucks dat hauls them seafood and stuff?"

"Not to my knowing. Why?"

"We know that she had a refrigerator truck and that Raymond Cloyd drives that sucker for her. Her truck broker in Houston done told the investigator as much earlier today."

"Let me say this: I've never seen a reefer rig around here with Mia's name on it," answered Alden wondering if indeed she did own a truck. After all her best friends were in the trucking business. Could she have had a big truck for a tax write-off of some kind, as much money as she made?

"I wondered about that when Cecil Bell told me awhile ago and thought I'd call and let you know ahead of time so you can go ahead and try to find out. This investigation is moving to Oakwood since two principals in this case are from Oakwood, Alden."

"I'll find out about the truck. You want me to call you back?"

"Hell no. You gonna be so busy answering dem newspeople's questions that you ain't gonna have time to call nobody. See you around," said John, laughing as he hung up the phone.

Elated at the progress he had made on the case, Cecil walked into his boss's office with the scoop on Cloyd. The Louisiana State Police Troop D of Lake Charles the with the city police and local sheriff's office quickly organized the sting. As a courtesy, Cecil was invited to come over to Lake Charles to help run the show and arrest Cloyd.

Cecil left immediately after changing back into his uniform, gassed up his cruiser, and left for the hour-and-a-half drive to Lake Charles. Abusing the taxpayers' property as he hammered on the solid white Crown Victoria, Cecil made it in fifty-eight minutes. The plan was to watch for Cloyd and Katy at the chicken coops (port of entry-scales) and keep them under surveillance until they bumped the docks at the drop point, and then pick them up. Cecil called the Texas DPS and asked that they keep an eye out for the truck, and it was all set up.

After Cloyd and Katy got off the Interstate 610 loop in Houston eastbound, Cloyd patiently worked his rig though heavy traffic. As they passed the Mount Belvieu exit on I-10 Raymond's CB radio announced that a black and white (DPS) had just rolled off the get on ramp and fell in behind his rig. A quick glance in the mirrors confirmed that indeed the trooper was running hard to catch up with him. He had been closely watching his speed. The recent change in the speed limits in the Houston area had dropped the speed limit back to 55 and 60 around the greater Houston area to reduce smog. The black and white passed a few cars and dropped in behind his trailer four car lengths back and hung there. Raymond watched for the dreaded blue lights to start flashing. It never happened. The trooper pulled to the shoulder and stopped.

Katy asked, "Wonder what that was all about, Ray?"

"Don't know. I ain't been speeding or nothing. Probably got a call on something more important than hassling truckers," answered Raymond checking his mirrors again.

Katy talked while Raymond pushed the big unit toward Lake Charles. At the Winnie entrance ramp another black and white fell in behind the big truck. It followed for a mile or so then passed Raymond's unit. Running another mile or so, the trooper pulled onto the road shoulder and stopped. Katy counted four more bears before they hit Beaumont. Raymond noticed that a Beaumont squad car followed them completely through Beaumont on out to Rose City.

Raymond told Katy that he was stopping in Orange to get something for his headache. He told her that he felt bad and needed some sleep. She agreed to go ahead and deliver the load. Raymond pulled into the truck stop and found a parking spot. Raymond closely watched the parking lot for a while as he rubbed his neck. Raymond had thrown his black cowboy hat in the bunk and put on a baseball cap before he stepped out the truck. Katy offered him some headache pills, but he refused them saying he wanted another kind. Katy moved over under the wheel, adjusted the seat, and drove away.

"That's strange," Katy thought as she pulled out of parking lot and stepped up on the big road. "He ain't never gone in a truckstop with a cap on since I've known him. That hat musta been causing his headache." Katy shrugged as she put the big rig up in the wind for Lake Charles. The Orange County deputy watching the parking lot in a white unmarked Ford Crown Victoria duly reported that the truck under surveillance was moving again toward the Louisiana state line, unaware that Raymond had jumped ship.

Raymond had stepped between the drive wheels and sleeper cab of Volvo parked next to his truck and stayed there until two drivers come along headed to the building. He ambled out from behind the sleeper cab and fell in behind them as they made their way toward the building. Raymond quickly went to a pay phone and dialed. He talked less than a minute and hung up. Raymond went to the counter in the restaurant ordered a cup of coffee and waited.

Twenty minutes later a tall, lanky teenage boy sat down beside Raymond and lit a cigarette. Raymond drained his coffee cup, paid for his coffee, and walked out to the front of the restaurant with the tall boy following. Raymond's eyes carefully scanned the area. Satisfied no one seemed to be watching as he got into the passenger side of a late-model Chevy Blazer. The boy drove out of the parking lot while Raymond scanned the whole area looking for a police car.

Satisfied that he had got out of the big truck undetected, Raymond told the boy to drive to Katy's trailer. As they approached Katy's trailer, the only police car they had seen was in Mauriceville. It belonged to the deputy who lived down the road from the Katy's trailer house. The deputy was cutting his lawn on a riding lawn mower as they passed. Raymond told the boy to come inside and help him put some stuff in the Blazer. Quickly gathering his clothes, boots, and other stuff, Raymond loaded everything in the back seat of the Blazer and left. He and the boy drove into Beaumont.

He went the bank. Raymond withdrew eight thousand dollars from the truck account Mia had set up for him. The banker offered his sincere condolences to Raymond on the demise of his business partner. Stunned and deeply hurt, Raymond let the man rave on about what a great woman Mia was. The banker told him that he attended her wake but was unable to attend the funeral. Raymond simply nodded, turned, and hurried out of the bank. On his way out town Raymond dropped the boy at a discount tobacco store, gave him a twenty-dollar bill, and headed east on I-10.

Katy had no trouble finding the produce dealer in Lake Charles. She skillfully spotted the trailer on the unloading dock. She opened the door and climbed down to check with the warehousemen when Sergeant Cecil Bell appeared out of nowhere. It was not dark. Katy had no idea how the trooper got to her door without her seeing him.

Cecil pulled Katy roughly away from the truck door as three more officers materialized and grabbed her arms and handcuffed her hands behind her back.

With his Glock pistol drawn, Cecil stepped up on the running board and peeked inside. The bunk curtains in the sleeper were tied back. As Cecil stuck his head around the high back seat, he realized that Raymond had done it to him again. The truck cab was empty. Cussing under his breath, Cecil picked up the black cowboy hat lying on the bunk.

Katy was hysterical by now. Not a single officer would talk to her. She was screaming obscenities right and left, sending every police officer in the state and their mothers to hell with her foul mouth. When Cecil walked up to her holding the black cowboy hat, she turned the blasphemous tirade off like a radio. Cecil, now mad as hell, asked, "Where is he?"

"He got out at Orange at the truckstop and went to the house to get some sleep."

"Where's the house?"

"My place."

"What is he driving?"

"Tan-over-white '98 Blazer."

"Texas plates?"

"Yeah."

"Registered in his name?"

"Yeah."

"Read her rights."

Cecil turned and walked quickly to his car motioning two of his follow officers to follow. Both officers were lieutenants with long outstanding careers with the State Police. Standing beside Cecil's cruiser, the officers quickly decided what each would do to commence the search for Cloyd. One officer would call the Orange County sheriff's office to get the license plate number on Cloyd's Blazer and check Katy's place. Another would notify The DPS to stop and arrest Cloyd on suspicion of murder. Cecil would get an APB issued in Louisiana and Texas for Cloyd.

Tall as a pro basketball player, the black Calcasieu Parish deputy had Katy standing by his squad car waiting for the word to stuff her. She had calmed down somewhat but was firing off questions to the officers standing around her. Characteristically, every officer ignored her. Knowing a big deal was coming down, each officer anxiously awaited for the three troopers to send them hunting Raymond Cloyd. Cecil was busy on the phone and radio getting help from all the surrounding parishes and counties. (Parishes are in Louisiana. Counties are everywhere else.)

When Katy got to the state line or to Lake Charles, Raymond knew all hell would break loose. It dawned on him that the law would soon know what kind of personal vehicle he owned. He needed another ride quickly to elude the dragnet that would be laid for him.

Chapter 14

Thirty-plus hours with no sleep turning the McAllen short turn, plus the news about Mia, left Raymond wrung into deliriant perplexity. Nothing in his hard-lived life unsettled Raymond like Mia's death. He'd vowed to tell her goodbye one last time. He remembered that tomorrow would have been her thirty-third birthday. Sobbing and talking to himself incoherently, Raymond remembered how he had begged her to leave that man alone. If she had just agreed to let her boyfriend or himself beat the dogshit out of Ryan, she would be alive today. He blamed himself for her death.

Turning into the used car lot off US 96 just north of Beaumont, Raymond Cloyd had seen better days. Feeling and looking like he had been rode hard and put up wet, he now really did have a headache. He finally accepted the finality of Mia's death. Raymond knew he was being hunted. He had correctly figured that with all the Texas police profiling and following his truck from Mount Belvieu to Orange that the Louisiana police would have been waiting at the state line to arrest him. Somehow, the authorities had figured out his involvement. If they arrested him in Louisiana instead of Texas, they wouldn't have to extradite him back to Louisiana. The need to change rides overrode his desperate need for sleep and rest. He knew if he didn't get some sleep soon, he would never be able to evade the massive manhunt for him.

Winford 'Monk' Monkhouse, owner of the car lot and a beer-drinking buddy of Raymond's, walked out to the Blazer when Raymond didn't immediately get out and come inside. The trailer house that served as an office and living quarters sat on the back of the lot with twenty-seven late-model pickups and SUVs lining the front of the lot.

Monk, nearly fifty-five, walked with a slight limp. A claymore mine had severed his left foot just above his ankle in 'Nam. Not quite six-foot tall, his slightly hunched shoulders and carefully styled gray hair lent dignity to his rugged outdoorsy cowboy appearance. He had dazzling brown eyes set under a broad forehead. Monk's mouth was set in almost a perpetual grin with perfect teeth. Dressed in a tan western shirt, starched Wrangler jeans, and plain brown leather roper boots, he was a true Texan to the bone. The prosthetic left boot perfectly matched the right boot, thanks to a friend in Houston in the business. Monk wore no cowboy hat but wore a handmade leather belt, bought from an inmate at Huntsville prison, that set him back over a grand with the gold and sterling silver buckle and matching conchos.

Monk loved the old ways his parents taught him. A man is no better than his word and that sort of stuff. In today's business world it is trite, corny, and laughable—in Monk's world, it is chiseled in stone. Living just on the edge, he knew the shortcuts, the easy way, and fine-tuned the questionable ways to accomplish a goal. He had been the sales manager for several high-end car dealerships in the area but taking advantage of the people who needed a little help buying some wheels galled him to no end. Monk fixed the problem. On this car lot Monk made the rules and a lot of money selling and buying pickups and SUVs.

Looking in the Blazer, Monk hardly recognized Raymond. "Man, what in the hell has happened to you?" asked Monk opening the driver's side door.

"Everything, by God. Worst week of my life, Monk," said Raymond barely audible as he turned to get out of the Blazer.

"Come on inside and get out of this heat and tell me 'bout it," said Monk.

"Man, I ain't got time to sit around and bullshit. I got to have another ride and get my ass out of here."

"In trouble with the law?"

"Yeah, they looking for me now. I ain't had no sleep in over thirty hours," answered Raymond.

"Get that ass on in the office. I'll be in there in a minute," said Monk looking up and down the highway before sliding under the wheel of the Blazer and parking it in a shop-shed building that he used to detail his vehicles before putting them up front for sale. Monk returned a few minutes later with registration and title he had retrieved from the Blazer's glove box and threw them on the desk.

"What kind of ride do you need, Ray? You see one out there you like, or do I need to find you something else?" asked Monk.

"A pickup will do fine. You got a good one that's ready to go, automatic, cold air, good tires and the works?"

"That four-door Lariat is loaded, low miles and nearly new. Just got it in. One of them big oil company executives had it on lease to pull his bass boat with."

"I don't like a solid white pickup."

"You don't want to be noticed, do you? Shit, nobody pays any attention to a white pickup unless the driver is messing up. Everybody will think it's a company-owned truck on its way to a job somewhere. This 'un is really nice."

"I guess you right 'bout that, Monk. Fix the paperwork."

"You not gonna ask what the difference is gonna be?" asked Monk incredulously, knowing that Ray was a hard trader. He sat down at his desk and begin the paperwork himself.

"You oughta be paying me boot, Monk, but I ain't got time to haggle."

"I'm gonna fix this where you can leave in thirty minutes with that pickup out there. I'll call and get your insurance transferred for you in the morning. Call me from somewhere and I'll fax you an insurance card. Give me a thousand dollars and I'll take care of all this business for you."

Raymond nodded and took a wad of bills out of his pocket and laid ten one hundred-dollar bills on the desk. Monk worked furiously on the paperwork, glancing up at Ray occasionally, knowing something was bad out of whack with Ray.

Monk got a set of keys from the board on the wall by the door that must have had fifty sets of keys hanging from little hooks and pitched them to Raymond. "Go on out yonder and start that sucker up. Let that air conditioner be cooling. That sucker is probably hotter than a pot of collards sitting out there in the sun."

Raymond found the pickup was as nice inside as his Blazer. The air conditioner was topnotch. Raymond backed the truck off the line, pulled it around in the back, and transferred his stuff from the Blazer to the pickup. When he drove back around to the office, Monk had the paperwork ready.

"Ray, if you need me, call. Be sure to get to a fax machine tomorrow, and I'll get your insurance certification card to you. I'll probably send that Blazer off to a car auction next week and get it out of here. Don't want folks asking too many questions," said Monk knowing pretty much that Ray was leaving Beaumont for good. Monk badly wanted to ask Ray about his problem but decided against meddling in his business. Shaking hands, Raymond drove out of Monk's car lot and out of his friend's life.

The sign read "American owned." Not a soul behind the third rate motel office desk could speak even passable English. Sitting back off US 96 out of Beaumont a few miles north, the motel sported a small oriental restaurant and nail salon in the motel office building. A row of twenty motel rooms, ten in front, ten on the backside of the main building.

A frail oriental woman of indeterminate age desperately tried explaining the room rates to Raymond as he checked out everyone in the lobby and behind the desk. His searching eyes found a an old man wearing a Texas Rangers baseball cap sitting near the door to the kitchen wearing a well-soiled white apron, probably the old woman's husband. A younger version of the old woman with most of her teeth stood behind the registration desk with the old woman. A well-dressed young Asian man stood in the doorway to the nail salon. Two teenage Asian boys watched from the dining room door as Raymond cased the place. A teenage Vietnamese girl sat watching TV and reading a book in the far corner of the lobby. Raymond guessed the girl to be around fifteen. As he approached her, she looked up and smiled. Raymond asked if she spoke English. "Yes, I do. How may I help you?" was the answer in perfect English.

Raymond quickly explained that he wanted a room and not register, a meal, and he preferred his room on the backside of the building away from the highway. For all of this he told her he would pay sixty dollars in cash. She motioned for him to wait and walked over and had a short conversation with the lady behind the desk. Returning she handed him a room key as she said, "Eighty dollars and it's a deal."

Raymond under any other circumstances would have haggled, but now, time was precious; he handed the girl a hundred-dollar bill and walked with her to the desk for his change. Raymond told the girl he was leaving most of his stuff in the pickup and it damn well better be there in the morning. She quickly informed her non-English-speaking American family of his edict. It was agreed that a careful eye would be kept on his pickup. To the astonishment of every one in the lobby, Raymond turned to the desk in word-perfect Vietnamese thanked everyone, ordered his meal, reminded them to watch his pickup, put both hands together under his chin, slightly dropped his head and shoulders, and walked out the motel lobby door to his pickup.

Chaotic discussion started, with everyone talking at once, when the young girl told her mother and grandparents that Raymond was wanted in connection with the Frappé Monsieur case over in Louisiana. The TV had shown a recent picture of him just before he arrived to rent a room. Like most American citizens born halfway around the world, the question arose if money was offered for information about this man. The young girl explained that she had not heard, but usually the law gave rewards for this kind of information in America. The Vietnamese grandparents were all for making money that wasn't worked for and told the younger children it was their patriotic duty to see that this man was apprehended. Intensity of the discussion rose to a fever pitch with the whole family talking at once and deciding how to get money from the law for information leading to the arrest Raymond. The young girl reminded them that in America sometimes it is best to keep quiet and let the law work it out.

No one noticed the lobby door open. Raymond stepped back inside and moved in close to the Vietnamese family all still talking at once. The old woman noticed Raymond first, pointing and backing up, fearing a massacre surely would be next for her family.

All bickering stopped. Raymond again called the young girl to the far side of the lobby. Explaining to her exactly what happens to folks that didn't tend to their own business in Texas didn't seem to phase her one iota. She just smiled and looked at Raymond, glanced over at her family, shook her head indicating negative, and turned and faced

163

Raymond and still smiling replied, "You will be perfectly safe here till morning, Mr. Raymond Cloyd. After daylight tomorrow you're on your own."

"That's much better, young lady. I'll be gone before sunup," answered Raymond, realizing that she knew his identity, "I'd like to have my food as soon as possible in my room, please," said Raymond turning to leave asked, "How do you know my name, young lady?"

"Your picture was on TV. You are wanted in connection with the frozen man in Louisiana," replied the girl. "You will be safe here till morning."

Staying close to home, Milt and Lea had gotten to be news junkies since Mia's accident. They watched every local news show and listened to every radio newsbreak on the local station. Lea was grieving for her friend and praying that the law didn't tie them to Ryan's death. Her nerves in the meltdown mode, her infidelity was gnawing at her conscience, and Sly was taking Aunt Mia's death much harder. Last night Sly told her that she never wanted to go shopping again. "If Aunt Mia is not there it won't be fun anymore, Mama. Why did this happen to Aunt Mia?" sobbed Sly as she ran out of the den to her room. Lea followed her baby and tried to console and explain why sometimes bad things just happened.

Especially quiet at her shop since that night in Lake Charles, Amber listened to the radio and the gossip in her shop about the frozen man case. No one had connected Mia and the Frappé Monsieur yet. Norris had badgered her constantly since that night to take her out. Amber finally told him to cool it for a while. Sam had his drawers in a wad because he was shut out also. Cool as Amber was, this last week had put some doubt in her mind and gray hair on her head. Lynn had promised to call, he didn't. She drove by his place a few times, but his big truck was always gone. It was time to do Lea's and Sly's hair. Neither one had called for an appointment. She had been thinking about taking off a couple days and driving down to Padre Island and lie around on the beach.

Lea's mother was in the shop today and told Amber that Roger could not find Mia's real father so that Mia's estate could be settled. Anna dropped by and said she hadn't seen Lynn in nearly a week.

Anna said that Lea had offered her a job but that she hadn't decided to take it yet.

Anna didn't know that Lynn and Lea were an item. Amber had kept their affair to herself knowing that if she got the chance to date Lynn, she was going to take it. Amber thought maybe she might just offer to take Lea or Anna with her to Padre Island.

One of the beauticians in Amber's shop remarked that she and her husband had slipped off down to Holly Beach for the weekend. Already dark complexioned, Amber remarked that she didn't need a tan. Laughing, the beautician said, "We went out on the beach for about an hour the whole time we was down there but we wore that bed out in the motel at Cameron. I bet I'm pregnant again."

"Is Holly Beach pretty nice and all?" inquired Amber walking to the door, turning the closed sign around, locking the door, and getting ready to sweep up.

"It's okay I guess. Didn't stay out there long. The motel was great but I'm not hard to please when me and my man can slip off a couple of days. Besides that, I don't have to be quiet when we're having sex. No kids around to wake up."

"You got the motel phone number in Cameron?" said Amber.

"Right here in my purse," answered the beautician already digging the phone number out for Amber. "You planning on going to Holly Beach?"

"Yeah, I'm gonna to take off a couple of days and get away."

"Dark as you are, you don't really need a tan, Amber."

"I need to some time away from here. Holly Beach is lot closer that Padre Island."

"Taking somebody with you?"

"Don't know yet. Might be another week before I go. Be nice to have a hunk to play with while I'm down there, though."

"Lynn Howard would be my choice if was going to slip off from my husband. He is the sexist man I know. He probably needs a woman to get his mind back right after Mia's death and all."

"Yeah, dream on," said Amber, "It's not likely that he's gonna go anywhere with me and besides that, what am I supposed to do, walk up to him and say 'Come on down to Holly Beach for a couple of days with me, you big stud'? I want to screw you till you can't walk."

"That's about what I would tell him if I wanted him to slip off down there with me."

"You are full of shit."

"Well, all I can tell you is not to sit around on your ass and do nothing. You heard Mia say that she asked him to take her to that cowboy thing out in Jasper, didn't you?"

"Yeah, I remember her saying that. But I don't know about just inviting him to go lay up and have sex.'

"They ain't a man alive that wouldn't jump at the chance to have that great-looking body. Hell, it even turns me on sometimes, and I ain't that way."

"Maybe you ought to try it sometimes. It ain't bad as you might think," said Amber as she slapped the beautician's butt and smiled.

Cecil stayed up late hunting Raymond. He finally got a room at a motel in Lake Charles and slept fitfully a few hours before getting up and leaving for Oakwood. He would talk in person to the sheriff and try to drag a clue out of him or find out what he could tell him about Cloyd. Cecil explained to Alden Malone that if Cloyd wasn't apprehended by noon today, the FBI would take over the investigation, which meant that Cloyd would probably slip through the net. Alden offered to show him Ryan's apartment and take him to talk to Roger Hart to see if he could shed any light on the whereabouts of Raymond. Sheriff Malone told Cecil that he wanted to meet with Roger Hart at the cemetery where Mia was buried, adding that Roger Hart knew more about Mia and her business than anyone. Mia had worked for Roger all her adult life, Cecil was informed. Cecil declined the opportunity to look at Ryan's apartment but opted for an interview with Roger Hart.

Just five miles out of the city limits, the ancient Methodist church, sitting under five huge live oak trees, was founded in 1859, according to the sign by the road. The stained lead-lined windows with biblical icons embedded in each windowpane were the cheapest sold when the windows were installed. More than a century and a half later, today— the windows were priceless art. The cemetery sat on the south side of the church surrounded by an antique ornamental iron picket fence. A large gazebo sat between the church and the graveyard fence. Small in comparison to the Catholic cemetery uptown, the Methodist cemetery's grounds and churchyard were nevertheless professionally kept. Burial was now open to only members of the church and their family. Mia's grave was the only fresh grave in the cemetery. All the wilted wreaths would be removed today when the grounds maintenance crew arrived.

Roger Hart had ordered Mia's tombstone (monuments are what the salespeople call them) the day after the funeral. Roger indicated that he wanted to be present when the monument was set. The monument people had come two days earlier and poured the pad for the tombstone. Roger made a trip to the cemetery to measure and make sure that Mia's headstone was not outsized, showy, or gaudy in the plain and simple graveyard.

Roger received the call from the monument people informing him they were ready to set the stone at his convenience. Arranging for a nine o'clock meeting with the monument crew, Roger then called Lea and asked her to come out to the cemetery and watch. Lea agreed to meet her dad at the cemetery. Roger did not call Mia's mom. Roger had correctly concluded that the woman had lost touch with reality in their last conversation. Roger and his daughter would meet at the cemetery and set Mia's tombstone and try to put this tragedy behind them.

Sly found out about her Mom's planned trip. Sly was dressed and ready to go when her Mom finished dressing. Lea, not having the heart to tell her daughter no, allowed Sly to go with her to the cemetery.

The late August morning, a carbon copy of the last few weeks, humid heat scorched the haze off the muggy air by nine o'clock. A white Ford one-ton flat bed truck with a overhead chain hoist rail carrying Mia's tombstone, a big dolly, a half pallet of sod, a wheelbarrow, shovels, and other miscellaneous tools was parked near the gazebo. The crew sat waiting under the gazebos drinking coffee and soda pop. Lea arrived a few minutes before her dad and sat in the Suburban with Sly until her dad arrived.

A white four-door Ford pickup sat near the cemetery gate. Lea assumed it belonged to the tombstone setting crew. Roger arrived shortly followed by the sheriff and a state trooper in separate cars. Roger waited until the sheriff and Cecil got out and greeted them with a handshake. Alden introduced Cecil to Roger. Lea and Sly got out to see what was happening. Sly listened to the men talk a minute, walked to the gate, and entered the cemetery heading to Aunt Mia's grave.

As Sly walked down the path toward Aunt Mia's grave, she paid no attention to the moss-encrusted tombstones. She realized that the man kneeling at Aunt Mia's grave wasn't part of the crew sitting under the gazebo. She watched him a few minutes until her granddaddy and Mom caught up with her. Deep in thought or prayer, the man kneeling at the graveside did not hear them approach. Sly looked at her mom and granddaddy. Both shake their head. Lea put her right fore finger to her lips for silence. The arrangement of flowers lying before the man on Mia's grave was fresh. Finally the man stood up, wiped the tears from his from his eyes, and put on his cap. As he turned to leave, he was startled to see that he had an audience.

Roger walked ahead and asked the man if Mia was of kin to him. His answer was a curt yes. He walked around Roger, Lea, and Sly towards the gate. Cecil and the sheriff were now approaching to the cemetery gate to enter. The man stopped momentarily then walked on towards the gate. Both men nodded as the bearded man walked by them. Roger called to Alden just as Cecil recognized the man. Cecil turned and caught up with the man as he unsnapped the safety strap of his holster, pulling his Glock pistol.

"Raymond, I have your hat in the car."

"How did you know I was here, Officer?" asked Raymond.

"I didn't. I come to pay my last respects to Ms. Comeaux," said Cecil.

"You know I got to take you in, Raymond?" said Cecil. "You are wanted for the murder of Sanford L. Brooks, also known as Ryan Roberts."

All four men walked to Cecil's squad car. Cecil got Raymond's black cowboy hat out and handed it to him. Raymond put the hat on and held the cap in his hand.

"Let me read him his rights," said Alden realizing that Cecil had in custody the most wanted man in America.

Sly and Lea stood back watching as did the monument crew. When Alden finished reading Raymond his rights, Cecil turned him around and cuffed his hands behind his back. Raymond offered no resistance. Sly walked up beside her granddaddy and asked, "Why are you arresting this man, Sheriff Malone?"

"He is wanted for killing Ryan Roberts, Sly," answered the sheriff.

"But he said he was kin to Aunt Mia?" Sly replied.

"Are you really kin to my Aunt Mia, mister?" Sly asked Raymond.

Raymond looked at the ground for a full minute. He finally raised his head, tears streaming down his cheeks and answered softly, "Yes. Mia is my baby. Mia Cloyd Comeaux is my daughter."

Chapter 15

Sheriff Malone called ahead on his cell phone to tell the dispatcher that he and Trooper Cecil Bell had apprehended Raymond Cloyd. Sheriff Malone thanked God that Cecil didn't call in on the radio. He and Roger Hart had unfinished business with Raymond before Cecil took him to Lafayette. When they got to Oakwood, Sheriff Malone didn't lock up Raymond immediately. To the surprise of everyone, including Cecil, he led Raymond into his office along with Cecil and shut the door. Sheriff Malone asked, "Cecil, would you remove your cuffs from Raymond, please?"

"Why?" asked Cecil.

"Raymond, Roger Hart, and the judge have some important unfinished business to tend to before you haul Raymond off. Roger and the judge are on the way down here."

"What kind of important business? That judge is not going to turn him loose. There is a federal warrant out for him. Kidnapping."

"Nobody's gonna turn him loose, yet. However, you probably gonna have to, sooner or later. If you can't find hard evidence in that truck of his, you ain't got jack shit against this man that you can go to court with. That's another story. Raymond is Ms. Mia Comeaux's daddy. He needs to sign some papers to get her estate and will closed and all. Mr. Cloyd here has just come into a helluva lot of money and some nice property, Cecil."

"Okay, but I don't want him to get up out of that chair," said Cecil, unlocking the handcuffs and indicating that Raymond take a seat next to sheriff's desk.

"Mr. Cloyd here was trying to avoid arrest. He will be charged under federal law."

"Bullshit. I didn't see the man trying to avoid anything, Cecil. He was grieving at his daughter's grave when I seen him. He never resisted us in no way. If you can't find blood that belongs to Ryan Roberts inside that trailer you and that coroner down at Lafayette are gonna have a hell of a lot of explaining to do about arresting a man that you just assume did something. I believe this man answered a whole bunch of questions the night you found Roberts over at the Butte Larose rest area. Why didn't you arrest him on the spot?"

"Where were you the day before we found Ryan Roberts, Mr. Cloyd?" asked Cecil.

Raymond looks at Cecil and never uttered a word.

"What's the matter, can't you talk or what?" asked Cecil.

"You just read me my rights. I choose to remain silent until I have a lawyer," said Raymond.

"Just answer the question, Cloyd!" screamed Cecil.

"I choose to remain silent until I have the lawyer of my choice with me," said Raymond.

"Your choice, my ass. You don't get to choose nothing," said Cecil.

"The hell he won't. Where'd you come up with that, Cecil? In a few minutes he will have enough money to hire the best damn lawyer in the country and pay cash up front," said Sheriff Malone desperately trying to move the investigation out of Oakwood and away from Mia. He had rued the day that he called Sheriff Miller in Lafayette to help him out. Sheriff Malone never imagined that this whole debacle would fall in his lap. He had figured out that Ryan's past couldn't be investigated without messing up a whole bunch of folks here in Oakwood.

Sheriff Malone's secretary tapped on the door before she opened it just enough to let the sheriff know that Mr. Hart and the judge were waiting to see Mr. Cloyd. The sheriff opened the door and invited the men into his office and closed the door. Mr. Roger got right down to business as he asked the judge what did they need to do to get Raymond's part of Mia's inheritance transferred to him. The judge told Raymond that if he would sign the papers Mr. Roger had, then the monies and properties would be transferred into his name.

Raymond signed, and Mr. Roger went to work getting Raymond's inheritance from Mia transferred into his name.

Mr. Roger informed Raymond that the big truck he was driving was registered in Mia's name, and it was now the property of Sly Myers, adding, "Before property or money can be put into his account this truck must be turned over to me in good shape. If you are found not guilty I'm sure Sly will work out something so you can buy the truck."

Raymond and Mr. Roger exchanged all the necessary information to get their business straight. Mr. Roger informed the judge that Raymond would have his money in the bank of his choice in a week, all this settled, and Mia's will executed. Somehow during the course of all their conversations everyone in the sheriff's office except Cecil began to feel that Raymond wasn't guilty of freezing Ryan to death but probably knew who did.

The judge asked Raymond sort of off the record if he could unequivocally prove where he was and what he was doing thirty-six hours before the time he was questioned by Trooper Bell at Butte Larose. Raymond told the judge, "Without a doubt I can, your honor."

"Any kind of lawyer will have Mr. Cloyd free before you can charge him," said the judge to Cecil.

"This man has murdered a man and you're talking about letting him go?" asked Cecil.

"If you can't put this man at the crime scene, which you don't know where that is either, how are you going to connect him to this at all? For all we know he was just being a good citizen. All he had to tell you that night was 'I didn't see anything' and that would have been the end of it," said the judge, looking at Sheriff Malone shaking his head.

"We going to try him here in the sheriff's office, your honor?" asked Cecil, now mad as hell about the way the tide had turned in Raymond's favor.

"No. But mark my word, when Mr. Cloyd gets his high-dollar lawyer over in Lafayette, he is going to make you, that Sherlock Holmes coroner, and the DA look like fools. He can afford a high-dollar lawyer tomorrow. I've kept up with this case real close. I want to know how you can make a kidnapping charge stick on a man who has told us that he can account for all his time. This man is a long-haul trucker. His time in the truck is accounted for on a federal document twenty-four hours a day in fifteen-minute increments when he is working," said the judge.

"What would be your advice then, your honor?" asked Cecil.

"You and the DA talk it over. You can't prove this man absconded. You found him at the graveside of his recently deceased daughter. His co-driver delivered the load he had on his truck. If you can get some DNA out of his trailer, you may have something on the man. Otherwise, you are up the creek. You go out and arrest a decorated Viet Nam war veteran grieving at the graveside of his only child with the assumption that he killed Roberts because he was a child molester. True, nobody filed charges on Roberts for child molestation, but a good lawyer could find at least four of Robert's victims right here in Oakwood. Right now, with the evidence you have, you'd be lucky to get this man convicted of carrying too big of a bible or singing too loud in church," said the judge as he got up to leave the sheriff's office.

"Somebody killed Ryan Roberts and dumped him in my jurisdiction, and I intend to find the man's killer," said Cecil.

"That's what you get paid for, Cecil but I believe you are whipping a dead horse here," said Sheriff Malone.

"I'm calling Lafayette and moving him over there," said Cecil.

"Suit yourself," answered the sheriff, getting up and indicating that the talking was over. Sheriff Malone was praying under his breath that Raymond would not implicate his dead daughter in this, therefore opening up a whole new problem.

Cecil put the handcuffs on Raymond again and led him out to the booking desk. The deputy at the Lafayette sheriff's office said they would have a car on the way to pickup up Raymond in minutes.

Lea, Milt, Amber, and Lynn decided to meet at Lynn's place after they found out that Mia's dad had been arrested for killing Ryan. Lea found out from her dad before the news really got out.

Mr. Roger called to let Lea know that Sly owned a big truck that had belonged to Mia and Mia's dad had been driving it. Mr. Roger told Mia that Raymond seemed like a nice man and the sheriff thought they were railroading him. As soon as her dad hung up, Lea called Amber and Lynn, telling them it was important that they meet and discuss something that had come up. Lynn suggested they meet at his place since it was sort of out of the way and more private. Amber agreed to be there. She hadn't seen Lynn since the funeral. He had not called as he promised. Anna said he seemed to be taking Mia's death harder than anyone thought. Lea finally called Milt and told him something serious had come down and they were meeting at Lynn's place for pizza, beer, and talk. Lea would take Sly to Mam Maw's house.

Due to the gravity of the fact that the man the police arrested was Mia's dad, a whole lot of serious questions were thrown out about this serious predicament they were all involved in. No one was eating pizza. What if Raymond talked and implicated all of them? How much did Mia tell her dad before she got him to take Ryan out of Norris's trailer and put him into his trailer? If Cloyd talked even a little bit they would all be in real trouble.

Amber, hardly eating, remarked, "If this Raymond Cloyd talks, he will implicate himself. A deputy told me a while ago at the shop that they may not even have enough evidence to hold him. At best, they would have one hell of a time proving he did anything, according to what he said the sheriff told them. If Raymond is smart, he will not open his mouth. I don't believe he will implicate Mia in this."

"I don't either. Dad said he seemed to be a great guy. Dad talked to him at the sheriff's office while they got everything straight about Mia's will. Mia's dad got three hundred thousand dollars in cash from Mia's will and some real nice property. He can and will hire a good lawyer. Dad told me basically what Amber said. They have no evidence yet to charge him with anything. Sheriff Malone said if they can't find blood or some kind of DNA match in his trailer they will have to release Mr. Cloyd," said Lea looking at each person at the table for a minute.

"Surely after they talked in front of him at Sheriff Malone's office, the man will know to keep that mouth shut," said Lynn.

"You'd certainly think he would," agreed Milt.

"You think Sheriff Malone and the judge talked in front of Raymond to save Mia's reputation?" asked Lea.

"Without a doubt they did. The law and lawyers never talk shop in the presence of an accused person," answered Lynn.

175

"And another thing that has worried the shit out of me since that night—," said Lynn looking at everyone at the table.

"What?" asked Milt and Amber together.

"How did Norris's trailer door get unlocked without jimmying the padlock? Somebody had to have a key or a master key or they got a locksmith out there. This has bothered me as much as the Stud Muffin getting frozen," remarked Lynn.

Lea and Milt spoke up at the same time; Lea giving the floor to Milt, "Lea and I discussed this twice before we found an answer, Lynn. Back when Mia bought twin jet-skis and a trailer to haul them on, she asked if she could park her big ski-boat trailer under our shed out at the shop until she could get her own boat shed built. We agreed, and she put her boat trailer under our long equipment shed out at the shop. We in turn gave her a key to the gate. That same gate key fits every padlock we have, gates, trailer doors, toolboxes, and all. I remember telling her that her key would unlock any gate or door we have a padlock on since we use identical padlocks on everything."

"She must have remembered," said Lynn shaking his head.

"Mia's bound to have tried the key sometime during all this ordeal to see if it would work," added Lea near tears.

"She could have rode by the fuel stop anytime Norris's truck was parked there and tried her key. This is not rocket science but if Mia did have a key made and give it to her dad I hope he has got rid of it before they arrested him," said Amber.

"Oh, we heard from another recording company today. That makes five so far that has called about Sly's CD that Toby mailed Monday," said Lea.

"What y'all gonna do 'bout the contract since Toby has skipped out on us?" asked Amber.

"Well, one guy has called twice and offered a standard contract without an agent clause, whatever that is. I don't ask because I don't won't to show my ignorance no more than I can help," said Lea.

"I say we ought to start looking for Toby just to satisfy Sly and fly him to Nashville. Let Toby negotiate a deal and you handle the money," said Amber.

"How will we find him?" asked Lynn.

"I guess start out by going down to the radio station and find out if they have heard from him," said Milt, "They tell me that all these dudes in that business keep in touch and are likely to know where to find him."

"I know one thing. That is one weird dude that works up at that radio station at night," said Amber looking at Lynn. Everyone laughed and the tension eased up some.

Milt got up and told everyone that he and Lea had a big day ahead of them and they were cutting out. "Call if you hear anything about Raymond."

Amber got up to leave. Lynn was at her side in a heartbeat. "I was hoping you might hang loose with me for a while, drink another beer, and talk," said Lynn as Milt and Lea went out the door.

"I got a long day myself tomorrow, but I might drink just one with you," said Amber, searching his eyes for a deeper meaning.

Lynn went to the fridge and got two long necks, popped the tops, and set them on the bar. He went over and turned on the CD player with some slow dancing music. He approached Amber and held out his arm. Amber slid right into his arms and they began to dance. She heard he was a good dancer—she had never danced with a man that was better.

Lynn was holding her closer and closer, rubbing himself on her. Amber rubbed back. She was the first to make skin contact by nibbling his neck. At this point the dancing sort of stopped and the kissing and feeling started. Amber stuck her tongue deep into Lynn's mouth as he unsnapped her bra. She looked at Lynn and smiled before she kissed him hard. Lynn led Amber around the bar into the hall to his bedroom. He never turned on the lights as he began to undress her. She was on fire for this man.

The next morning one of the girls in the shop noticed Amber walking funny and asked her if she had a problem.

"Yeah, I do. A big ole problem. Gonna get some more of that problem tonight," said Amber grinning. "I stayed over at Lynn's last night. Didn't hardly get no sleep and I'm so sore I can't hardly walk. It's so bad I'm going back tonight for some more of the big problem."

All the girls laughed and high-fived Amber.

Lea had just put another record company executive off for a few days until Milt decided if Toby could be Sly's agent. Milt had to make up his mind or the frenzy might die down. Lea phoned Milt on the job telling him that she had just talked to another record company guy and how anxious they were to meet and see Sly perform. Lea told Milt that the guy pointedly asked if Sly had an agent or business manager. Milt promised to call her back in an hour to let her know if she could start looking for Toby and sign him up as Sly's agent. Lea knew he was going to call Paw and her Dad before he made his decision. She knew what the decision would be because her dad had suggested that she sign Toby up and get started making records and money. Paw always agreed with her daddy so Lea picked up the phone and called Wendell Carr, the radio station owner.

Wendell knew that Ryan and Toby had cut a CD for Sly and in fact told Lea he had a copy of it on his desk. Lea asked if he knew where or how to get in touch with Toby. Lea explained why they wanted to contact Toby and offer him a job. Wendell assured Lea that he could find Toby if he was working or trying to find work in the radio broadcasting business. May take a day or two but every effort would be made to find him Wendell assured Lea.

"Sly talked to your evening DJ last evening and asked if he had heard from Toby. The man didn't say no and wouldn't elaborate. That might be a starting place, Mr. Carr," said Lea.

"That sounds good to me. Let me call him. I'll keep you informed. If I do find him and your plans don't work out, I plan to offer him a job as station manager and I'm going to retire. I haven't been feeling good lately, Lea. Talk to you later. Bye," said Wendell.

Sly sat on the corner of her mom's desk asking, "Think we can find Toby, Mama?"

"We gonna sure try, baby. The radio people network pretty good. Mr. Carr said that it might take a couple of days but they will find him," answered Lea, fingering a couple of stray hairs back into place on Sly's award winning haircut.

"Mom, I been thinking about something."

"What's the matter, baby?"

"You know school starts Wednesday. Since today is Monday and Amber is closed today, do you think that me, you, and Amber could go shopping for a few school clothes down in Beaumont and maybe eat lunch like we used to on Saturdays before Aunt Mia died?" asked Sly.

"I don't see why not, baby, if we can find Amber. No telling where that heifer is, but we'll find her. You ready to go?" asked Lea knowing perfectly well that she was.

"Yes ma'am."

"You call Amber. Here are her numbers. Sometime she goes down to the shop on Monday morning to do some bookwork. I'm going to slip into something and put some makeup on."

Amber had had her second cup of coffee and a shower when Sly called. Amber had not been home long. Sly didn't know where Amber had being sleeping the last couple of nights.

Sly asked, "Mama and me are going to Beaumont shopping for me some school clothes and I want you to come with us if you can."

"I ain't dressed yet. Y'all wearing shorts or jeans?"

"Shorts. We'll be over there in thirty minutes. Okay? See you," said Sly hanging up, delighted that Amber would agree to go with them shopping. Sly knew her mom always needed help buying clothes. Sly or her mom didn't own a stitch of clothes or shoes that Aunt Mia didn't approve of. Sly wanted Amber to go because she thought that Amber would be less conservative. Sly was about to find out that Amber dressed more conservatively than Aunt Mia or her Mom and was a better shopper but also a lot of fun to be with.

Just before the girls got into Beaumont, Lea's phone rang. Lea put the call on the speakerphone. It was Cleve Loe, the night DJ at the radio station in Oakwood. Amber recognized him instantly as the guy that started every sentence with "like."

"Wonder what that little jerkoff wants with yo mama," Amber whispered in Sly's ear.

"Mrs. Myers, my boss Mr. Carr, asked me to call you and give you Toby Nichol's telephone number. It's like," said Cleve as he gave Lea the number twice.

"See what I told you?" said Amber out loud, making Sly start giggling. "That little fart can't talk and yet he calls himself a radio announcer. Where Wendell Carr gets these folks from, is what I'd like to know." asked Amber barely above a whisper making Sly laugh out loud.

"Mrs. Myers, my boss told me about Sly and her record contract and all. Is Sly gonna like have herself a band, like a regular country and western band, ma'am?" asked Cleve.

179

"Well Cleve, that's something we haven't thought about. Why?" asked Lea glancing at Sly whose head was shaking vigorously, yes.

"Please call me Cleo. Everyone else does. Well, like, I play the keyboard and piano. Could I like audition for a gig with Sly? Like her keyboard man, Mrs. Myers? I can also read and write music," announced Cleo.

Glancing over at Sly and Amber, Lea slowed her Suburban down replying, "Yes, you can audition, Cleo. My dad, Sly, and Toby if we can get him to come back and work for us will have the final say so about the band members. Sly will probably be a superstar before Christmas according to what they tell me. Do you play well enough to be in a superstar's band, Cleo?" asked Lea, looking over at Amber. Surprising Lea, Amber was nodding yes along with Sly.

"It's like I never had the chance to play big time, so that is why I am just asking for a shot at the job. I think you will be pleased with my talent, Mrs. Myers. And like, thanks. You know where to find me when you're ready," said Cleo hanging up before Lea could say bye.

"Well, Sly welcome to show business. That's the first of a million calls similar to that you will be getting," said Amber as she cracked the door window and fired off a cigarette. "You know that turd head Cleo has done listened to that CD of yours probably at least a hundred times and probably got a copy of it at home. What I'm saying is that in my experience with these kind of folks like Cleo, music is all he cares about. If he has the balls to ask for the keyboard job, you can bet your ass that ole Cleo can tote the load. I've seen 'em like him before. That little fart ain't even learned to talk yet but I'd bet they ain't none no better on a keyboard and I ain't ever heard him play a note. I bet he's got the arrangement already fixed for your big song, Sly," said Amber taking a long drag off her cigarette.

"You would think we would have thought about a band by now," said Lea. "Milt called just before we left and said it would be okay to find Toby and hire him as Sly's manager. I'm going to pull over in this parking lot and call this number and talk to him now if he's there," said Lea slipping the big Suburban into a parking slot in a mini-mall parking lot.

"Yes. He is here," the receptionist at the radio station in Prescott, Arizona replied. "Hold, please."

"Hello. Toby Nichols. How my I help you?" Toby asked politely.

Lea was a tad nervous about tracking Toby down, then calling him. She knew Sly wanted this man to help her but he left after Ryan came up missing. Would he hang up on her or accept her job offer. "Hi Toby, this is Lea Myers, Sly's mother. How are you doing?"

"Getting by, Lea. How about you and Sly?"

"Doing great. I called to offer you the agent's job. I have the paper work signed and notarized. All six recording companies have contacted me and are interested in signing a recording deal with Sly. Are you interested in the job?"

"Yes, but I can't take it,"

"May I be so brazen to ask why not, Toby?"

"You aren't brazen, Lea. The simple fact is that I'm flat broke and don't have a car anymore. I'm stuck right here until I can get on my feet. Sorry."

"Let me ask you again in a different way. If I make all those problems leave immediately, would you catch a plane to Nashville, take care of Sly's business, and then fly back to Lake Charles. Someone will pick you up at the airport."

"Yes. Yes, indeed. I would be honored to be her agent."

"Can you cut them loose today? Right now would be better. I know that ain't the way to do business, but you do need to be in Nashville tomorrow morning."

"I can leave in two hours."

"Give me your whole name, social security number, and driver's license number and state. I will call and get you a car rented and delivered to where you are now. In Nashville, you can take care of the car rental. When you get the car, go to the closest bank or big truck stop and tell them you want to cash a Com-Check. I will deposit two thousand dollars in an account in your name and you can write checks on it at any bank or truck stop that cashes them. Your airline ticket will be waiting at the airport. We use Delta. Go to a cell phone dealer like AT&T and call me. You need a good cell phone. We will put the phone on my credit card. Use this credit card number until I can get you one in your name. Call me in an hour," said Lea, giving Toby her cell phone number. "Anything else?" she asked.

"To talk to the recording company executives I will need a copy of the agent's contract to show that I am authorized to do business in Sly's name. Also a paper stating that you give me approval to do business in her name since she is a minor and you and your husband sign and date this and fax it along with the contract."

"I will take care of that. Anything else?"

"Yes, Thank you so much. You will never regret giving me this once-in-a-lifetime break. Thanks again and tell Sly thanks for me."

"You are most welcome, Toby. Hurry home. We have a band to get together. See you soon. Bye."

"Yeah, I know. See all of you soon. Bye."

"Let me drop you and Amber off at the mall and I'll make all these phone calls and find you inside. Boy that is load off my mind that Toby is now on our payroll and them folks can quit calling the house."

"Mama, can we take some of the insurance money from Aunt Mia's wreck and buy Toby a nice car? Sort of like a company car until he gets on his feet? He should be making lots of money before long. We got that little house down close to the radio station Aunt Mia left me. Toby could live there for now."

"Yes, baby. That's fine with me if it's okay with your Pa Paw Hart."

"I'd make a play for that boy when he got back down if I didn't already have me a man," said Amber trying to act serious.

"Who you dating?" asked Sly.

"Baby, I been seeing Lynn the last couple of days. I believe we may have us something going for real. I'm 'bout ready to get married, have some kids, and settle down."

"You mean getting married to Uncle Lynn?" asked Sly.

"Yeah, when he is ready. Lynn is really changed lately, I guess he's ready to settle down." said Amber glancing over at Lea.

Lea just bit her lip and never said a word. Amber noticed that the news about her and Lynn was not well received. Amber didn't care. She had Lynn and intended to keep him.

Chapter 16

Toby made it back to Oakwood Thursday with a great recording contract. The record company executives were coming Saturday to interview Sly, her mom, and dad. They knew she could sing, but Toby felt they needed to meet Sly, Sly's parents, and grandparents and understand that they could work with these folks.

Lea and Amber, with Anna help managed a great meal and party for the record company executives. Two men and a woman came to check out their newest talent. Sly's outgoing personality and ability to carry on a conversation with grownups smote the men. The woman, brought along especially to find something wrong with Sly and her folks, admitted later that she might be the ideal teenager. The executives knew within an hour that they had discovered the mother lode. They intended to mine it.

Sly and her mom had arranged to have the house she owned near the radio station furnished and the utilities turned on before Toby got home. Anna, Sly, and her mom, had it fixed up looking great when he got home. Sly asked Anna to come by once a week and clean up after Toby since he would be busy. Anna, coyly making her move on Toby, came over every time Sly and her band practiced at Toby's place. Anna quickly became Toby's assistant and friend.

Toby's skill in selecting the band members for Sly rivaled the best in the business talent wise. A pretty petite young woman from Orange, Texas, won the fiddle-playing spot. Getting the bass guitar job, from Dry Creek, Louisiana, a tall lanky young man left a great bar band for the job. Sly's drummer was a talented redheaded and freckled-faced young man, Randy Lefleur, a senior at Oakwood High. Her lead guitar player was a grown man Toby's age from Camden, Arkansas. Toby knew him from another radio station job and as a lead guitar player in a local rock band in Camden.

Playing that steel guitar exactly like Paw wanted it played had left this position in want. Paw insisted the steel player be extremely talented and not a copycat player. Paw insisted on innovation. Most of Sly's songs would be new, and the steel guitar would be the dominant instrument opening most of her songs. Finally, a timid young guy with slight speech impediment showed up wearing a bread company uniform and steel guitar setup that looked well on its way to a dumpster. Paw knew the man's daddy after talking to him. His daddy was paralyzed from a stroke. Tee Ray, as the young man was known, took to playing around with his daddy's steel guitar and was now playing with a bar band over in Winnie. He was single and going to trade school at night taking a course in air conditioning repair and maintenance. Reluctantly, and only because of his daddy's reputation, Paw allowed Tee Ray to set up and audition. Paw and Toby were tired of listening to folks who couldn't play well and with no musical creativity. They needed a talented steel player badly. In six weeks they were going to Music City to cut a CD.

Paw asked the band to play a chorus of Sly's new song and Sly would sing. Tee Ray would listen. When they stopped, Tee Ray would wait a minute and then start to play his own steel guitar intro version to the song and play on through with band.

Sly played her guitar intro and she sang one chorus and stopped. Everyone watched Tee Ray sitting behind his daddy's ancient steel guitar with his eyes closed, his callused hands beating time to music that had stopped, and his head and shoulders still moving in rhythm with his hands. He opened his eyes, looked at Sly, grinned, and winked. His hands hovered over the strings. Tee Ray kicked the intro off, his expert rendition completely catching every band member off guard from what they were expecting to hear. He kept playing. They all just stood with their mouths open and watching, then started playing along with Tee Ray, not believing what they were hearing and seeing. Tee Ray looked up at Paw when Sly began singing. The both-thumbs-up and smile from Paw inspired Tee Ray. Drawing from deep within himself and putting his extraordinary natural talent into playing the steel guitar got him the gig. He would quickly become known as one of country music's best steel players. The bread company would have to find another deliveryman.

Cleo, after a single short audition, got the keyboard job. Amber was right: Cleo had his own musical version of Sly's big song written when he was hired. The band's talent jelled quickly. Sly and Toby moved to make her band have that unique sound. Cleo just stepped up and assumed the bandleader role. Realizing Cleo's talent, Toby, Paw, and Sly just told him what they wanted and how they wanted it to sound. Cleo made it happen. Toby realized they had a band talented enough to play for the best in the business.

Sly had to give up her cheerleader position. Her new career was demanding on her time especially on the weekends. She would miss a week of school when she and the band went to Nashville to record a CD. Toby asked Lea if Anna could go with them to Nashville. Lea said it would be all right with her if it was okay with Lynn. Lynn agreed if her brother would come over and feed his horses and Bo while he was on the road. Milt decided to stay home and run things. Fooling everyone, Paw announced that he was going to Nashville with them.

Using Lea's and Paw's Suburbans and renting a small moving van, the convoy headed to Nashville. Toby volunteered to drive the small moving van with Anna riding with him. Amber promised Anna that she would help her brother keep an eye on things at Lynn's and might just stay out there if Lynn was gone on a run.

With a new CD made in just five days, the caravan left Music City Saturday morning on the way home. Sly's single was released two weeks later. The song went straight up the charts to number one in a week. It was approaching the top of the pop charts a week later. Sly's dream was half-true now.

Late in November during the Thanksgiving holidays, Toby arranged for Sly to open a concert for one of Texas's own and most successful country singers in the business. In Beaumont, Texas, the concert was a sellout in hours after the tickets went on sale.

Sly had sung a few times at special occasions locally but not in a concert. Thrilled to get to open for one of her favorite male singers,

Sly was getting ready for her debut performance working her band hard and practicing every spare minute. Toby assured Lea and Milt that Sly would be a sensation. The concert people gave Toby a wad of tickets for Sly's family and close friends. Sly's grandparents and dad were the first to get tickets then Lynn and Amber; Anna, Amber's girls at the shop got two tickets each. She gave her band members two tickets each and saved two tickets until later.

Sly's grandfather Roger Hart told Sly that he had sold the big truck to Raymond and he would pay her out by the month. Raymond's lawyer had the charges dropped when no DNA showed up. It never would show up. Raymond was using a loaner trailer that afternoon and night. His trailer was in the shop with a leaking compressor seal. Sly asked for Raymond's phone number and Roger gave it to her. She decided to call Raymond and ask him to come to the concert.

Raymond agreed to meet her granddaddy Roger out front and he would have the tickets for him and his lady friend, Katy.

The lights dimmed in the huge auditorium as a murmuring hush fell over the sellout crowd. The DJ from the local country and western radio station stepped into the spotlight to introduce Sly. Praising her talent and band, he told the crowd that his station was one of the first in the nation to play her current hit song and was proud to introduce the newest country music star in the land. As he pointed to the darkened stage a small spot light fell on Tee Ray sitting behind the finest new steel guitar money could buy. Tee Ray introed another song on Sly's album with a lot of steel-guitar work in the song. Pandemonium broke out as the crowd roared, nearly drowning out Tee Ray's perfect intro.

The big spotlight washed the dark away instantly revealing Sly in all of her beauty and poise with her guitar. Everyone in the back stood to get a better look, and then everyone stood as Sly began to sing. Lea and Amber were frantic, afraid all the screaming and hollering would distract Sly. Far from it, Sly liked this; it was even better than she ever imagined it would be.

Dressed in a black custom made western style bell-bottom pants and black western shirt with the yolks trimmed in off white showed her perfect body without making her appear older than she was.

Enjoying herself beyond anything she had ever done Sly had six songs to sing, saving her number one hit till last.

Before Sly started her last song, she walked to the edge of the stage and looked in the first row at her dad and grandparents, Uncle Lynn, the girls from Amber's shop and Raymond sitting next to her Pa Paw Roger. Walking to the edge of the stage was never rehearsed and had the stage manager puzzled. Sly, smiling her killer smile said, "This song I want to dedicate to my godmother, Mia Comeaux who was killed in a car wreck recently. I know she is watching. Thank all of you for the great support," stepping back to her spot and nodding to Tee Ray. The moment Tee Ray began to bend them strings the already standing crowd began to clap with the beat of Randy's drums.

Standing beside Lea and Amber off stage in the wings, the star of the concert had watched Sly and her band perform flawlessly as seasoned professionals. He touched teary-eyed Lea on the shoulder and said, "Lea, I know how proud you must be of Sly right now. She is the most talented young person I've ever met. Shortly Sly will be the best known and most recognized singer in the world. Trust me. Your world as you know it is changing as I tell you this. I wish all of you the very best," as he patted her shoulder and left to get ready for his act. Any other star would have been in a snit for being upstaged, but not the president of Texas. He was rich and famous and not the least bit insecure as most entertainers are and he felt great about helping Sly launch her singing career.

When the song ended, Sly encored four times. Walking off the stage the last time Sly hugged her mama, shut her eyes, and said aloud, "Mama, dreams do come true."

The End

About the Author:

Born and reared in Dubach, Louisiana, Don finished high school then attended Louisiana Tech University leaving to get married. Working on a large farm from age twelve, he learned to operate heavy equipment and drive big trucks. Having been around trucking for over thirty-nine years, qualifies him to use the trucking industry as the background setting for this novel. Don spends his days off writing from notes made while working. He plans to make that last run in August '03 and devote most of his time to writing. He does plan to do some limited part-time driving just to stay in the game. Don's hobbies include reading, writing, hunting, and fishing.

www.ingramcontent.com/pod-product-compliance
Lightning Source LLC
Chambersburg PA
CBHW020411290526

45785CB00002B/513